The MAGIC of BIG LOVE

Getting Comfortable with Uncertainty

SHEILA
PEARL

http://www.agelessandsexybooks.com/
info@SheilaPearl.com

Printed and bound in the United States of America
ISBN: 978-0-9967865-1-5

Cover Painting: Tara Diamond
Back Cover Portrait: Elizabeth Gramm

Contents

Foreword

There are so many things in life that we don't understand — or, more correctly, don't remember that we *do* understand. One of these things is that every one of us has the ability to communicate with that aspect of The All that I call *God*.

Yet, it goes beyond that.

This ability to communicate *soul-to-soul* is not limited in any way. People the world over who are deeply in love have found that out, as one person begins a sentence only to have the other end it, or as one holds a thought only to have the other speak it.

Must we be "deeply in love" to connect and communicate with each other in this way? I believe the answer is yes. Yet the term "in love" should here be defined.

By being *in love* I am not referring to merely or only that state of mental and physical ecstasy that we call Eros, or romantic love. When I use the term *in love* I am referring to a state of existence in which we are enveloped, submerged, utterly and totally immersed in another; a state in which there is virtually no experience of separation — mental, emotional, or even physical. The sense of "you" and "another" disappears, and the only sense that is left is of "us."

The Greeks taught us that there are three kinds of love — Eros, Philia, and Agape — the first being an erotic, sexual kind of love; the second being a familial, brotherhood kind of love; the third being a very elevated, unconditional kind of love wanting only the very best at all times for all others: what is often call God's love. What I am referring to here is *all three at one time.*

The only way that I can describe such a state is by using the term *Oneness*. The experience is at once one of ecstatic union and blissful detachment, intense excitement and total calm, ultimate *givingness* and penultimate *receivingness*.

In this remarkable state — which, incidentally, is not as impossible to reach as its description may suggest — the ability to communicate back and forth with the object of such love is a given. Indeed, the *love itself* is a communication. Yet can one, even using the tool of *Perfect Love [Big Love]*, actually communicate with a person when verbal communication is, for some reason, out of the question? The astonishing answer is yes. And now comes this remarkable book by Sheila Pearl to prove it.

This text provides two gifts simultaneously. First, evidence that what I have said above is true. Second, the sweet wisdom that such an experience can provide. Taken together, we have here a gem of spiritual insight and a source of wonderful comfort for any person, but especially for those who are moving through the most challenging and difficult times of life.

In order to give us these gifts, Sheila Pearl has had to reach into her supply of emotional openness and share of that with uncommon generosity. That she has done, and for that I am personally grateful, for by doing so she has brought us messages that open the mind, heal the heart, and connect the soul with its Larger Self.

It is from this larger perspective that we are allowed to see the blessing in every human moment — including those moments when we may be overwhelmed by a feeling of separation and loss in the face of a beloved other's serious illness or death. How do we deal with such crises? By what manner or means can we spiritually discover, much less embrace, their purpose? With what tool can we hope to find peace?

With this tool, right here.

I am going to suggest to you that you have found this tool either because you need it, or you know someone else who does. Turn these pages, then, with anticipation and gladness. I believe you will find that it is good that you are here.

— *Neale Donald Walsch*

Prologue

The discipline of blessings is to taste each moment,
the bitter, the sour, the sweet and the salty and be
glad for what does not hurt. The art is in
compressing attention to each little and big blossom
of the tree of life, to let the tongue sing each fruit, its
savor, its aroma and its use.

– Marge Piercy

As I complete the manuscript for this story, I am 76 years young and bold. This story is true, although I have changed the names and done what is necessary to protect the privacy of the people who are central to my life and are included in these pages.

I have written this story to read like a novel; it is a continuation of the journey of "Stella" which began in the first book of the *Ageless & Sexy* series: *The Magic of Sensuality* — *a love story.* I created "Stella" to be an *everywoman* character: Stella is you, and Stella is me. In this second story in the *Ageless & Sexy* series, Stella's transition and discovery process is mine — and may also be yours. This is a story of the emergence of what I call *"Big Love"* both within myself and with others.

Throughout this story, there are elements of *magic* and *Big Love*: for me, *magic* is what happens when imagination and an open heart meet any challenge in life. For me, *Big Love* is how I experience myself when I face my fears and dig deep for courage as I move forward toward my own possibilities. For me, *The Magic of Big Love* allows me to say *YES!* to life as long as I have breath.

When I was serving my congregations in Franklin Lakes, New Jersey and Newburgh, New York as cantor and co-spiritual leader, I sang a full-spectrum repertoire of songs and liturgy. One of my favorite Israeli composers has long been Naomi Shemer who is famous for songs like "Jerusalem of Gold" and "Al Kol Eileh" ("For All These Things"). The message of the latter song is central to the theme of this story:

Every bee that brings the honey
Needs a sting to be complete
And we all must learn to taste the bitter with the
sweet....
Bless the sting and bless the honey
Bless the bitter and the sweet...

Whatever age or stage you are in your life, it is inevitable that you face uncertainty. The fundamental law of the Universe is uncertainty, which is where possibilities reside. Life is about change. Life is about possibilities. Life is about growth. Life is about movement.

This story is about my own journey in getting comfortable with uncertainty. During many times in my life, I directed the majority of my focus to resisting change and protecting myself from the discomfort of uncertainty. When I began to accept uncertainty as a fact of life, when I began to trust that the Universe did in fact "have my back," I began to lean into the many challenges and difficulties I have experienced. Leaning into the challenges is a practice, like meditation; you are never done learning how to lean into challenges, you just learn to lean *deeper*.

I have integrated much wisdom from being a singer throughout my life: I've learned to breathe deeply from my belly, not allowing the fears and anxieties I am feeling to tighten me and constrict me;

I've learned to smile regardless of the tragedy or pain I am facing; I've learned to stay present to my life even when I would often much rather fall asleep or distract myself from difficulties; and I've learned to never give up — to keep going even though I want to quit — and to complete singing my song.

In the works of Esther and Jerry Hicks, one of the many rich messages from *Abraham* best describes what "Big Love" is about:

In your resistance you get tired, and so, you need
rest.
And so, you go from resistance to rest to resistance to
rest.
But what about rest to eagerness, rest to passion,
rest to alignment, rest to clarity, rest to brilliance?
You can get this Energy moving within you and
when you are up to speed with that Energy,
you are clever, you are fun, you are full of vitality;
your timing is good!
Then you are living life as you intended.

I have discovered from my personal experiences and my work with clients over the past 40 years that the greatest barrier to living life as you intended is *fear.* Fear can stop each of us from stepping into our magnificent selves, can thwart our creativity, and can block our access to courage and compassion.

I have learned that the key to opening the doorway to our most delicious lives is *vulnerability.* When we allow ourselves to be vulnerable, open, and authentic, we invite our greatest possibilities to flourish and experience ourselves as *Big Love.*

It is only when I lean into uncertainty, trust that the Universe has my back, take that deep belly breath as I lean into my fear, and

— with conscious intention — open myself up to courage that I experience profound joy and lightness of spirit.

Many years ago, in the midst of the "hell" of my dear husband's dementia, I learned to ask big questions about life. Questions which changed the quality of my life: "How can I make this difficult situation a blessing?"

In my 76 years of beautiful life so far, I've been to the top of the mountain many times, and I've been in the depths of the valley many as well. I've suffered the death of my infant daughter, two of my stepchildren, my parents, my grandparents, my friends, and my husband. I've prevailed through my own journey with cancer, depression, and addiction. I've navigated multiple careers ranging from being a school teacher, opera singer, psychotherapist, cantor and spiritual leader, educator, speaker, and now a life coach specializing in relationships and life transitions. It has been a rich and sweet journey in which the bitter and the sour have been an integral part.

As I remind you in each chapter: "Stella is you...Stella is me..." This is my story and this is also your story, wherever you may find yourself. I have written it so that you may find yourself in a dialogue, a situation, or a valuable quote which I've carefully chosen as part of the tapestry of this story.

May you find in these pages and in this story some wisdom and guidance that will assist you in getting comfortable with uncertainty, for it is in the uncertainty of life that your greatest possibilities reside.

— *Sheila Pearl*

1

Being Present

Life invites us to get in touch and stay in touch with
our soul. Living your life from the place of soul can
tell you many things that living your life from the
place of mind and body alone cannot.

— Neale Donald Walsch

STELLA: I'm imagining how I can stop time.
ME: What does it feel like to stop time?
STELLA: I feel that magical oneness, like time is
            standing still.
ME: When have you felt like that?
STELLA: When I am in love…
ME: How do you know when you're in love?
STELLA: When I feel that we are one…
ME: What does that feel like?
STELLA: That we created "us" — I'm not separate.
            I'm not alone.

Stella is you…Stella is me. Stella was at a turning point, facing
uncertainty about her finances, her living situation, and her desire
for a romantic relationship. She had just completed her morning
meditation and stretching exercises, sipping her coffee. Her little
voice whispered, "Read your mail!" She looked at the mail which
had been piling up on her kitchen counter.

As she sorted through the envelopes, she was puzzled when she saw several letters from law firms. One by one, she opened all six envelopes. They were letters from lawyers in her area, offering her their services for saving her home. *Saving my home?!* She had *no idea* what these letters were about. After looking into the situation, Stella discovered that the bank which held the note for her reverse mortgage had filed a notice of foreclosure with the Court.

Stella felt a surge of electricity rush through her body. *What am I going to do now?* Stella was in default of the terms of her reverse mortgage. She wasn't paying attention to her financial obligations. She had not been paying attention to her mail. She had neglected to pay her real estate taxes on time. The bank was taking action.

I'm going to be homeless! she thought to herself. She felt fear taking over her entire mind and body.

She called her attorney, who reassured her that he would represent her, and asked, "Are you able to make a deal with the bank?"

Stella was not in a financial position to make any deal with the bank. They wanted $244,000 for a property that was assessed at $116,000. She asked her attorney to buy her as much time as possible to vacate the property. He assured her she would have several months. Fear became Stella's constant companion.

Fear shouted, "You will be homeless — on the street!" while Stella practiced her usual response to fear: "Thanks for sharing."

Stella shared her situation with a friend who suggested they plan to rent a house together. It seemed like a good idea; she was weary of living alone and looked forward to sharing her beautiful possessions with someone else.

Her friend encouraged her, "I would love for you to bring your piano and beautiful dining room furniture!" Stella wanted her treasures to be appreciated; she longed to be a part of a household again. "We can have dinner parties and music, music, music!" The thought of creating a household, hosting dinner parties and enjoying music together filled her heart with joy.

"We can have a Passover Seder and invite all our friends! It will be wonderful!" Stella was excited about the possibilities of a future "family of choice" in which she could re-create the kind of joyful moments she once created during her marriage.

As Stella looked around her apartment, she realized that her beautiful dining room table and chairs, china closets filled with crystal, porcelain statues, and fine china had been taking up space in her home being unused, gathering dust. They were physical reminders of happy times during her life with Adam before he became ill. These possessions represented Stella's soul connection with her loved ones, reminded her of all the times she experienced being **in love**. *In love* with her life. Feeling at one with her life.

As Stella was ruminating about her beautiful dining room set, she remembered the first Passover Seder in their new townhouse 25 years before that moment. Stella felt the tears welling up as she felt a sadness fill her body. As the images, aromas, and physical memories flooded her body, Stella felt grief overwhelm her as she acknowledged losses: her husband, many members of her family, plus the family gatherings, her cantorial career, her financial abundance, and her feeling of wholeness. Stella longed to feel in love.

She remembered that Passover Seder, reflecting on how excited Adam was when their new dining room set arrived, delivered in time for the holiday. The new china closets gleamed with glass and light, creating an elegant environment for their first Passover Seder in their new home, welcoming 35 members of their family.

Stella's joy in their new home was that there was room for children and grandchildren to sleep in the guestrooms. Stella was filled with anticipation as she set the tables with her fine china and crystal, stepping back to assess the beauty of her new blue linen tablecloths and napkins. She had been preparing the food for days; the aroma of the chicken soup wafted throughout the house. Adam placed the individual copies of the *Haggadah* on each place.

As Stella's home filled with members of her family, she felt a wonderful sense of *oneness* as each took their place around the large tables which filled the dining room space. Her home was filled with *us*. She felt enveloped by *givingness* and *receivingness* in the midst of that holiday celebration. There was no time. Time stood still. Everyone was totally engaged with the story in the *Haggadah*, with the holiday songs including *Dayeinu*, with the tastes and fragrance of the variety of festive foods, and with the hugs and laughter of the evening that filled the house with joy — a depth of joy for Stella that went straight to her soul.

Once everyone had either gone home or were tucked in for the night in the guest rooms, Adam and Stella sunk into their loveseat in their room. "It was a gorgeous Seder, bubbeleh…thank you," Adam said to Stella as he cuddled on the sofa next to her, leaning over to kiss her.

Stella's memories were commanding center stage. She remembered her first kiss with Adam, when she was 29 — then she remembered her last kiss with Adam, when she was 63. Those 34 years were filled with uncertainty and possibility, those kisses were magical moments for her; she felt time stand still. That first kiss ignited their three-decade marriage. That last kiss had a quality of eternity. She wondered, *How can I make time stand still?*

In her late 50's during Adam's illness, Stella had developed a daily routine that began with meditation; getting present. She experienced time standing still when she meditated. She began each morning with two big questions: *Who do I want to be today?* and

What energy do I want to bring into my space today? It took intention and focus. It always began with her breathing — her deep breathing.

Stella had been a singer all of her life, learning from an early age about the importance and benefits of deep belly breathing. Her mother and father, both singers, taught Stella how to breathe deeply: "Let the air come into your belly slowly and fill you up, without your chest getting tight, my darling." Stella associated deep breathing with loving her body, like a massage from the inside out.

Stella looked around her apartment, beginning to assess which items she would keep and which items to let go. She had begun to save money for the big move while she and her friend began their search for the best house to rent.

As Stella faced the immanent move out of her apartment, her daily routine of meditation became more challenging: she struggled to stay present. Her mind toggled back and forth between the past and future, mourning her losses then thinking about possibilities. Her body was feeling the effects of overwhelm.

As she looked around her 2-bedroom apartment which contained 45 years of acquisition — all six large closets and drawers in multiple dressers and cabinets were packed full of her belongings — she began to grasp the magnitude of her move. "I need at least six months to purge and pack!" she repeated, like a mantra. Days and weeks passed, and Stella was stuck. Although she was excited about the future, the picture she had in her mind about the work she was facing stopped her from taking action.

"Be present!" her little voice whispered.

Stella began to breathe deeply, leaning into her fear. "I can't do this!" was her voice of fear. "Thanks for sharing," she shouted in response. *Who do I want to be today?* Stella wanted to be courage and possibility. She wanted to take action.

"Be present!" her little voice shouted.

2

Do I Go?

What shape waits in the seed of you to grow
and spread its branches against a future sky?

— David Whyte

STELLA:	Should I go to meet him?
ME:	What would stand in your way?
STELLA:	The expense. I really don't have the extra money it would cost to go right now…
ME:	Money is energy. It's an exchange. I'm wondering what the real obstacles are…

Stella is you…Stella is me. Stella was excited; she had an unusual opportunity to finally meet Wally in person. Wally and Stella had connected on Facebook and discovered they had a great deal in common. They had agreed to become *Agape* friends — dedicated to loving one another in a very *Big Love* way: caring about one another on a soul level.

Wally had been invited to speak at a conference in California, not far from where Stella had been born and grew up. Stella still had friends and family in and around Laguna Beach, and Wally's conference was just an hour south. He invited her to join him at his favorite little B&B on the beach. If she made the trip, she would have the experience of hugging and kissing Wally at long last…something she missed and longed for. If she made the trip she would visit her friends and family as well.

What was the obstacle? Money. Stella was getting ready to move out of her condo into a house with a friend. The move was going to be expensive. She was intent on being financially responsible, to save her resources for rent and moving expenses. She was also intent on living in the moment and taking full advantage of every opportunity to connect with the people who mattered most to her.

She decided to see the choice as a matter of both/and, rather than either/or: by going to California, she was seeing the golden opportunity in front of her face. She was being present to her possibilities. She was also economizing in every way; her friend was giving her a place to stay in Laguna Beach and Wally had invited her as his guest at the B&B. Wally also wanted to pay for her car rental so that she would have the convenience of driving to and from the conference and B&B. Her expenses, aside from airfare, would be minimal.

"Everything you want is on the other side of fear."

Stella decided to go. She made her flight reservations, when she needed an additional $300 in her bank account. She had 24 hours to take advantage of the low airfare. "I think the Universe has my back…" she mused.

3

The Kiss

When you reach the end of what you should know,
you will be at the beginning of what you should
sense.

— Khalil Gibran

STELLA:	I felt his kiss in my sleep.
ME:	And…?
STELLA:	It was like a warm blanket around my heart.
ME:	And…?
STELLA:	I didn't want to wake up…I didn't want to face reality.
ME:	What is reality?
STELLA:	That he's gone…that no one kisses me like that these days…that I miss that feeling of the warm blanket around my heart.
ME:	I see you're focusing on what you DON'T have.
STELLA:	I'm feeling sad, empty, and alone.
ME:	Remember Adam telling you he would never leave you?
STELLA:	Yes…I remember. I think I'll meditate.
ME:	What happens when you meditate?
STELLA:	I connect with Adam.

Stella is you…Stella is me. As Stella was planning ahead for her trip to California, gathering the items she wanted to pack, she was also looking around her apartment, feeling a nostalgia as she saw her belongings with fresh eyes. She was facing pictures, furniture, hanging items, and household items that reminded her of Adam and her life with him. The large blue and turquoise ceramic vase they bought together in Jerusalem summoned her memories of their many trips to Israel. She was facing a big change in her life; she knew that moving out of her apartment — whenever that would take place — would be a big turning point for her.

Stella had been widowed over a decade and missed her husband's kisses. Adam had been her safe haven and her soulmate. Before he passed, Adam promised her that he would never leave her. She understood that he was saying that their love was eternal and that he would be eternally in her heart, even though his body died.

Eighteen months before Adam's passing, Stella began to connect with him by going into a meditative state, communicating with him, heart-to-heart, spirit-to-spirit. She had learned a specific form of spiritual presence called *"Kything."* During her *kything* meditation with Adam, she not only sent him her intuitive messages; she also received messages *from* him. When Stella first began these intuitive connections, hearing his messages, she wondered whether or not she was making it all up. While she was often incredulous, she continued to listen. In those conversations she was experiencing a *oneness* and a sense of *us* which felt like bliss. She felt no separation between herself and Adam: it was a timeless experience of *oneness.*

Adam challenged her: "When you think of me and when you're in my room, focus on the part of me you know is eternal; move away from the focus on my illness and your judgment of dementia…when you look at me, what you see is not me; what you feel in your heart is me."

During the several years of Adam's progressive illness, as he became less and less available to her, Stella had been angry with God and the Universe. Stella's teachers repeated over and over again: "Everything is happening **for** you, not **to** you." That was a hard one for Stella. She believed that dementia had stolen her husband from her. She felt alone, sad, and angry with her circumstances. "I can't swallow that the Universe has my back!" she shouted at the moon.

In Adam's messages, she heard, *"I know you're angry and feel like a victim. Imagine what it would be like to step aside from feeling that all of this was happening* **to** *you. Imagine that there's a blessing in all of this. Keep asking the question, 'How can I make this a blessing?'*

"This epidemic of dementia is an opportunity for people to experience new dimensions of awareness: family and friends are invited to see their loved ones in ways that bypass the physical and cognitive limitations this illness imposes. Teach others to be more present to their loved ones who are wrestling with dementia. It is important that friends and family approach the person with dementia on a more energetic and spiritual level. They don't have to have a typical conversation; they can simply be present. Teach others how to kythe!

"Embrace the wonder of everything…we are all one…we are interconnected with everything there is. Be curious and stop judging your situation. Love is all there is."

Stella mused, *Love is all there is…really?* She wondered about fear and anger. For her, they were real and visceral. She realized that she was judging her situation; she was angry about what felt unfair that Adam was basically "gone" and not "there" for her. Then she wondered, *Is what I'm experiencing in these conversations with Adam real?*

The gift of Stella's *kything* meditations with Adam became a fundamental part of her daily practice as she moved forward in her life after Adam passed. *Kything* became a basic technique Stella practiced for getting present and connecting with her clients and loved ones. It became a spiritual practice that led her to *Big Love*.

Love is all there is... she mused. *If Love is all there is...it must be big...very **big**.*

4

Belonging

People are starving for love, not knowing their heart is a magical kitchen. Open your heart. Open your magical kitchen and refuse to walk around the world begging for love. In your heart is all the love you need. Your heart can create any amount of love, not just for yourself, but for the whole world.

— Don Miguel Ruiz

STELLA:	I just want to belong...
ME:	Belong to whom? To what?
STELLA:	To that special someone who wants to belong to me.
ME:	How do you already feel you belong?
STELLA:	Well...I do feel I belong when I am with my Grace community, my speaker tribe and a few good friends.
ME:	I'm hearing a "but..."
STELLA:	Yes — but it isn't the same as when you belong to that one special person in a more intimate committed relationship.
ME:	You've experienced that kind of belonging. What is it you miss most about that?
STELLA:	The way my lover looked at me; I felt seen and cherished.

ME:	What else?
STELLA:	The way my lover kissed me with those tender little nibble kisses that said, "You're delicious."
ME:	I hear you…

Stella is you…Stella is me. Stella was wrestling with relishing her independence while also missing being in love. She enjoyed her friends and communities. She also felt an emptiness as she longed for tender intimacy. "I want those tender nibble kisses!" she would shout to the moon, and sometimes confess to her friends.

It had been nearly two years since Stella had let Matt go; she was on a mission to find that special someone; a man who could give her more than Matt was able to give. She was often tempted to invite Matt back into her life, as she remembered their delicious encounters. Since breaking up with Matt, she had begun to dread dating, wondering if it was too late for her to find a partner. She had briefly met with a few men who were not for her. Returning home after these dates became a painful ritual of Stella vowing to herself, *I'd rather be alone than with him!*

I'd like to be enough for me… she mused to herself. She thought of a quote which kept playing in her head, like a song: *Whatever you want from someone else, give it to yourself.* She wondered how that works when what she wanted was for another person to see her, to cherish her, and to give her tender kisses. As she sat musing on her conundrum, she replayed her memory of the last time Matt kissed her, nuzzling his face in her neck, then teasing her with little nibble kisses she could barely feel on her lips. He always left her wanting more.

Stella felt her body tingling as she remembered what she was missing.

Is my body telling me something about my soul? Stella wondered.

"I'm not defined by having a partner or not," she told her best friend. Yet…that tingling sensation was information. "I refuse to beg for love…that's ridiculous!" she shouted.

Everything is energy… She decided to transform her longings and tingling sensations into a larger scope of energy. She asked herself, *Who do I want to be today? What energy do I want to bring into my space today?* The singer in her came out to clarify what was happening. She remembered what it felt like to hit the high notes and bring a piece of music to life so that others would feel the poetry and melody in their souls. It was exhilarating, and her body vibrated with excitement when she accomplished her mission. Likewise, when she was in the "zone" speaking before an audience, and she felt that she had connected with them as she was expressing an idea, her body tingled with high energy.

"Use your energy and enthusiasm to love others, to love the world…" her little voice whispered. "It's all within you, all the time! It's the *Big Love* you were born to be." As Stella integrated the elements of *Big Love* within herself and applied the principles in her work with clients, she began to experience the reality of **being in love** with herself, with members of her family and her closest friends and clients. While her longing to **be in love** with a significant other continued to inspire her to remain open to that possibility, she was also enjoying *Big Love* with herself and the people who were central in her life.

5

Doppelganger

You are all messengers. Every one of you. You are carrying a message to life about life every day. Every hour. Every moment.

— Neale Donald Walsch

STELLA: I think I just connected with my "doppelganger."

ME: That sounds almost magical…tell me more.

STELLA: It's like my alter ego, my other self, a partner in learning and evolving.

ME: Where did you learn about that?

STELLA: First, Adam told me about parallel dimensions then I was attracted to learning more about that and heard about doppelgangers. Fascinating!

ME: How is your doppelganger helping you?

STELLA: Writing…writing things I've never written about before.

ME: So your doppelganger can support you in evolving your own creativity?

STELLA: Yes. It's always there. The doppelganger helps me bring it out into full view.

Stella is you...Stella is me. Among the many messages Adam brought to Stella during their *kything* conversations were his descriptions of what he had been discovering during his supra-conscious travels throughout parallel dimensions.

While Adam was sharing this information, Stella was often feeling dizzy and confused. She had never heard about these concepts and distinctions before her intuitive conversations had begun with Adam. After a few of their initial conversations, she began to do some research and learned more about quantum physics, parallel dimensions, and doppelgangers.

"You know where I'm going when I appear to be somewhere else?" Adam asked Stella. Stella was curious and wanted to know more. "I'm traveling to other dimensions. I know it looks like I'm gone, out of it, not with you, out of my mind. Part of that is true. I'm literally out of my limited mind and in the realm of supra-consciousness, jumping into parallel dimensions of consciousness, connecting with my doppelgangers." Stella sat motionless at times, as she listened to Adam's messages, wondering if she was losing her mind, as he talked about jumping into other dimensions. She listened and kept her heart open, as incredulous as she often was.

"How can I believe what you're telling me? It feels like I'm losing my mind sometimes, and when you talk about jumping out of your mind into other dimensions, I'm not sure if I'm not just going out of my mind and grasping at straws to connect with you." Stella wanted to believe. She also wanted to maintain her own sanity. What was Adam talking about when he mentioned connecting with his "doppelganger"? It was all so strange and almost surrealistic for her.

Adam urged her to keep her heart open, to keep listening to his messages, and to remain curious and open-minded about the ideas he was sharing. She agreed.

In the midst of their conversations, Adam taught her how to summon her doppelganger. She knew she wanted to write books but didn't know how to do it and she wasn't sure she had the talent to write. Once she connected to her doppelganger, she began to write with more confidence; she created a writing team and took action on fulfilling her dream to write and speak in the service of others.

"You can accomplish anything you can imagine," Adam reminded Stella. "Anything."

6

Bless Your Mess

Even in the darkness it is possible to create light.

— Elie Wiesel

STELLA: My life is such a mess!
ME: The mess is your message.
STELLA: What the heck are you talking about?!
ME: Whatever your mess is, that's your clue to
            what your life's journey is about.
STELLA: Like my financial mess is my life's message?
ME: Yes...
STELLA: Like my pain in my hip is my life's
            message?
ME: Yes...
STELLA: What about all those people who have
            everything they want? Whose lives are
            easy-breezy???
ME: Things aren't what they seem — everyone
            has something that's messy...

Stella is you...Stella is me. Stella has struggled with issues of money throughout her life. It had been a pattern. A problem. A challenge. A mess. Regardless of whatever else was going well, somehow her relationship with money was a constant thorn in her side (a pain in her hip?), a predictable problem to be solved.

As Stella was leaving the ATM and saw that her business account was overdrawn by $217, she was thinking, *What a mess! I can't cover my account's overdraft...more fees!* She was constantly fighting the voices in her head shouting at her: "You've been so stupid and short-sighted about **money**...what's the matter with you?!" She practiced telling her inner critic to back off, or would shout out loud, "Thanks for sharing!" and laugh.

She was well aware of how she had messed up financially: she made a disastrous choice about her life insurance vs. Adam's life insurance policies that years later would impact her quality of life in epic proportions.

"What was I thinking?!" Stella would often shout at the moon. She had to cancel certain insurance policies once Adam could no longer work: she made the fatal error of canceling Adam's large life insurance policy while maintaining her life insurance policy. While her motives were noble – wanting to protect Adam in case something happened to her – Stella's choice was disastrous for her, who had zero protection for herself once Adam died.

Once Stella retired from serving her congregation, she had no income except Social Security and whatever client fees she would earn from her work. She decided to take advantage of the reverse mortgage option, thinking she could save money and live in her condo indefinitely. In theory, it seemed like a good idea...until...

Until Stella's client fees dipped and she got behind with taxes and maintenance fees. Once Stella was in default of the reverse mortgage terms, the bank could call the note; eventually they did and Stella knew it would be inevitable that she would be required to vacate the premises.

Stella's challenge was to take total responsibility for her results without beating up on herself for her results. *Life is happening **for** me, not **to** me,* she continued to remind herself. She repeated: "The

Universe has my back..." Stella continued to ask the big question: *How can I make this challenging situation a blessing?*

Stella made a list of some of her answers to that big question. Because of her need to make a living from her professional work, Stella was constantly motivated to create something new, to persist in her networking endeavors, to defy the commonly accepted notion that people retire at 65 or 70. Stella did not see retirement as an option she wanted; she loved her work and felt grateful that she could wake up every day and work with her clients. Because Stella felt an imperative to function at a high level daily, she was highly motivated to take care of her well-being: she was dedicated to taking her supplements, drinking her greens, and eating healthy. She was in good health as a result of remaining vigilant on how she took care of her body and energy. Stella couldn't afford to get sick. She could only rely on herself to take care of herself. That was something she saw as a blessing!

7

Uncertainty

Life is eternally functional, adaptable and sustainable. Change is an announcement of Life's intention to go on. Change is the fundamental impulse of Life itself.

— Neale Donald Walsch

STELLA: I feel like there's no certainty in my life at all!

ME: It's a law of the universe that possibilities are infinite.

STELLA: How does that law help me?

ME: Embrace uncertainty; that's where possibilities exist.

STELLA: My feelings of uncertainty are so uncomfortable.

ME: Growth happens outside of your comfort zone.

STELLA: You're full of these little nuggets of wisdom and you're driving me crazy!

ME: It's important to "go crazy" on a regular basis…

Stella is you…Stella is me. Stella was standing at a crossroads in her life, feeling the uncertainty of every aspect of her life, personal and professional. Her head was spinning and she sometimes felt like she was losing her mind as she sought ways to manage her energy in the midst of the unsettling elements within each arena of her life.

She wondered how she could know whether or not her new living situation would work. Stella understood that living with another person could be risky business. She thought she knew her friend well, although she knew that it was true that you don't know someone else until you live with them. She knew from her work as a relationship coach and family therapist that this was certainly true! As excited as she felt about the next chapter in her life, she also felt some apprehension about the uncertainty in her future.

Stella wondered, *How will my new coaching program and next book affect my practice and her speaking career?* After all the work on designing her new *Big Love* life-education program and continuing to write her *Ageless & Sexy* books, the results on her income stream remained uncertain.

Stella had learned to expect that just as she was facing her own demons, the Universe would send a client who was struggling with a similar issue. She recognized the synchronicity and perfection of each so-called coincidence: the Universe had her back. Each of her clients had become her teachers and her mirror.

Stella's client, Jason, 45 years her junior, called her to ask for a coaching session: "I can't sleep at night! Everything in my life is like a bowl of Jell-O — nothing is certain. I don't know where I'm going or what I want to do next about my career. Help!"

Jason was Stella's reminder that everything is connected, that she was interconnected with everyone and everything in life. Age didn't matter; she was in her mid-70's and Jason was barely 30, yet they were both being invited by the universe to embrace uncertainty.

When Jason came in to Stella's office for his session, he hugged her with the 20-second hug Stella had taught him. She held him tight, knowing the power of that hug.

"I already feel better!" Jason exclaimed. They laughed together, knowing the magic of the long hug, appreciating the magic of their heart-centered connection.

As Stella was preparing Jason's coffee, she turned to him with a smile, "Fasten your seat belt, my dear — it's this uncomfortable uncertainty that you're feeling right now which is opening the doorways to more possibilities for you! Lean *in* to that uncomfortable feeling…"

Jason sipped his coffee, looking deeply into Stella's eyes, "Why does it have to be so hard?"

Stella smiled and took a deep breath. "What have I taught you about the 'Why' question?"

Jason laughed and revised his question: "How can I make this challenge matter for me?"

Stella leaned in to Jason, "That's more like it!"

After Jason left Stella's office, she meditated on the question, *How can I make this challenge matter for me?* She leaned into the silence and waited for the messages to flow to and through her.

8

Broke

The words you speak become the house you live in.

— Hafiz

STELLA: I'm frightened about being broke...
ME: What is the fear about?
STELLA: Not having enough money for basics...
ME: What are the basics?
STELLA: Food, shelter, car, office rent, phone...
ME: What if you could tell yourself that there is nothing you need?
STELLA: That seems crazy.
ME: Just try that thought on for a while...

Stella is you...Stella is me. Stella had been "broke" many times. Stella had also generated much abundance throughout her long life. She was experienced in making money and losing money, having money and not having money. Regardless of the money she had in her bank account, Stella was still Stella. What difference did the money make? What was Stella's truth when she experienced being what she called "broke"?

Stella remembered the day that Neale Donald Walsch said something to her she didn't understand: "There is nothing you need."

She looked at her teacher as he spoke these words and let them wash over her like a warm shower. Neale, who had become Stella's teacher and friend, had once been broke, unemployed, living in a tent, and foraging for food in dumpsters. Neale was an example of someone who transformed his life from being "broke" to becoming a best-selling author and global spiritual teacher. Every time Stella said to herself, *I'm broke!* she thought of Neale, and changed the words she was speaking to herself.

Stella shivered, thinking about being homeless, about foraging for food in dumpsters. Her little voice whispered, "You will never be homeless…there are too many people who love you."

She felt a comforting reassurance that it was true: there were several people she could count on if she were to find herself homeless and so totally broke that she needed a hot home-cooked meal and a safe place to stay.

"The Universe has your back." Every time Stella doubted that truth, she would notice how often, at those very times when she was running low on cash, a friend showed up to invite her to dinner or take her to lunch.

For someone who had spent a lifetime taking care of others – congregants, children, mother, husband, clients and friends – Stella was seeing that the truth of "what goes around comes around" was applying to her. Was Stella broke? She chided herself, *Notice how you talk to yourself…*

Stella realized that she had abundance in a variety of forms: clients who came to her for help, compensating her in exchange, friends who enjoyed her company and invited her for meals and gave her gifts, creative energy which she used to write books and develop new programs for her clients and audiences.

Am I broke? she asked herself again. *Absolutely not! I'm just a little short on cash from time to time.* She then began writing a chapter for her next book.

9

Abracadabra

(English translation from the Hebrew: "It will be created in my words")

Positivity is the gateway to possibility.

— Bob Luckin

STELLA:	It's too late for me!
ME:	Who made that decision?
STELLA:	The Universe.
ME:	Sounds like a big lie to me.
STELLA:	Seems true to me!
ME:	Only if you keep repeating those words…

Stella is you…Stella is me. Stella was afraid. Afraid of the clock. Afraid of aging. Afraid of not having enough. Afraid of not being enough. Her fears were blinding her. She couldn't see what was in front of her face. She couldn't see what was on the other side of the veil of darkness cast by her fears — until…

Until… she decided to lean into her fears.

Until… she began a daily discipline of meditation, gratitude journaling, and setting intentions for each day.

Until… she began to experience that her fears were an illusion and were also invitations to her to dig deep for the courage within her — the courage which was there to open her heart and her eyes to her own strength, creativity, and possibilities.

Stella's daily routine began with getting still: meditating on the questions that matter. Questions like: *Who do I want to be today? What energy do I want to feel today? What gifts do I want to give others today?*

Stella created a new book. She faced her fears with each word she wrote, with each chapter she completed. She began to feel the freedom she gave herself when she invited courage and compassion to replace the fear and judgment which had become constant companions.

She began a new women's group, inviting women to embrace their magnificence: The Ageless & Sexy Goddess Group. Each week, the "Goddesses" began with a "brag" — a way of acknowledging themselves for something they each felt good about, so the circle of women could celebrate one another.

It was Monday night — Goddess Group Night — in Stella's office. The women begin arriving at 6:45, meeting starts at 7:00, and often Stella is putting out additional chairs for late comers at 7:15. The Goddesses began with their "brag."

Hannah began: "I restrained myself from killing my husband when he bought a new car without consulting me!" Everyone applauded Hannah for her restraint as they laughed together.

Jodi continued: "I said yes when Adam asked me to marry him!" Amidst squeals and whistles, everyone applauded and circled Jodi with a group hug.

Loni was sitting quietly with tears in her eyes. Stella urged her to speak. "My dog Sophie died over the weekend...I'm a mess but came here tonight anyway." Each woman got up to gather Loni in her arms.

When the circle of brags was completed, Stella added hers: "I've dedicated myself to completing my next book and attracting my next life partner, however long that takes! I've already completed 42 chapters of the book and I'm making room for the one who is seeking me!"

The Goddesses applauded and shouted, "You go girl!"

Stella began the conversation by asking each woman to make a statement of what she believes is true about herself.

Hannah declared, "I'm strong and resilient".

Jodi added, "I'm lovable and blessed."

Loni and the others added their statements as Stella took notes. "You all understand the magic of your words, right? What you speak out loud matters."

Their conversation was animated, as each of the eight women shared with one another the self-limiting words they often speak to themselves, like "it's too late for me" or "I can't live my dream" or "I'm not lovable" or "I can't trust him." They challenged each other, helping one another to revise their self-talk.

Stella confessed to the group the many times she had said "it's too late for me" to herself (and others) when she was writing her recent book. She shared how she got stuck on completing the final manuscript on her first book as she was saying repeatedly to herself and her editor "I can't do this!" and her editor and coach kicked her butt, not allowing her to give up on her dream to complete that book. She changed her self-talk to "I'm doing this!"

10

The Big Lie

The sticks, the thorns, the leaves, the rain...
none of those have failed the rose.
They have only shaped and guided its blossoming.

— Ann Albers

STELLA:	I have believed a Big Lie all my life!
ME:	It sounds like you have discovered a truth about yourself.
STELLA:	Yes. That Big Lie was the reason I made every choice up to now
ME:	So now...since you know there was this Big Lie, what's the Big Truth?
STELLA:	I'm enough. I've always been enough.

Stella is you...Stella is me. Stella lived decades of her life believing she wasn't enough. She was driven to be more: more perfect, more accomplished, more successful, more famous. Then Stella discovered the truth of *Big Love*: she was already enough. She was already perfectly imperfect. She felt a heavy weight lift off her shoulders. She could breathe more deeply and freely. She felt an exhilaration when she could teach others how to let go of the Big Lie.

Ella arrived for her first session with Stella. "I've been holding onto your card for months! It fell out of my wallet last week and I knew it was time to call you..." Stella explored with Ella where she was coming from, what her challenges were, and what it was that brought her to this moment.

"I've been to hell and back in my relationships. Divorce. A long friendship that wasn't passionate. A passionate relationship that isn't really the relationship I want." They discussed in detail what Ella wanted.

Then Stella asked Ella the most important question: "What do you believe you can have?"

"I don't know if I can have what I want. I've never had it. I'm over 50 and don't know what it's like to have a deep and passionate love with a man. Maybe it's not for me..."

Stella invited Ella to envision the relationship of her dreams. "Allow yourself to feel the energy of what it's like to be in that relationship you want." Ella confessed feeling awkward imagining something she had never experienced before. Stella reminded Ella that she HAD already experienced the feelings she wanted to have with the right partner. "You experienced passion and pleasure with your lover. You experienced cherishing with your son and mother. You experienced a safe close friendship with your good friend. Now combine these into one person. Imagine how that feels."

Ella started to laugh, "It feels so weird and good...is it possible?" Yes...*Big Love* is possible.

Ella told Stella about her recent devastating experience with online dating, which had become her obstacle to going back online to meet possible partners. "I had reached out to this guy who responded, 'What makes you think I'd be interested in you?! You're ugly!' I began to question everything about myself. I began to wonder what my lover had seen in me. I began to doubt that anyone would find me attractive or want to be with me for **me**!"

50

Stella was stunned. She was looking at a woman who was beautiful from the inside out. Ella was grace and elegance personified. She explained the value of mirrors. "Sometimes we encounter people who are the opposite of what we are so we can get very clear about who we are."

Stella explained that we often meet people who trigger us to doubt ourselves, and when that happens, that's the moment we ask, "What's true? What's the Big Lie here?"

Ella thought of her lover who gave her the experience of feeling sexy, beautiful and desired. Her son and mother both gave her the experience of cherishing and being cherished. Her friendships were mirrors: she saw that she was valuable and lovable. "I'm going to practice feeling all of that...I'm going to remind myself every day that I'm enough."

Within a few weeks, Ella gathered the courage to go back online and allow herself to date a variety of men. She was learning to value herself and not take others personally. She was learning to see others as mirrors: some of them were distorted mirrors. Others were clear. She was noticing feeling liberated from the Big Lie. As the truth of who she really was became clearer to her, she enjoyed the adventure of dating more. "I believe that Rumi is right when he says that whatever I'm seeking is seeking me. I have a feeling he's nearby..."

11

Life Is

I would love to live
Like a river flows,
Carried by the surprise
of its own unfolding.

— John O'Donohue

STELLA:	The way my body is aging seems so unfair!
ME:	Interesting that you see something natural as "unfair."
STELLA:	I know, I know — the metaphor of the flower that blooms then withers…
ME:	You don't see the blossoming as unfair do you?
STELLA:	No…that's the beautiful youth of life, the vitality, the vigor…
ME:	Let me guess…the withering is to you the unfair part?
STELLA:	Yes. The inside of me still feels like the blossoming flower. It's startling to me that when I look at my aging body, I see the withering taking place. I don't feel like my spirit is withering….

Stella is you...Stella is me. There were times that Stella accepted her aging process with grace and ease. At other times, she resisted the fact of her aging, and felt angry and frustrated. At one moment, Stella acknowledged that she was ageless and sexy. In the next moment, she was focused on her aging skin, her physical challenges. Stella replayed her own words from a speech she had just given:

> *Who we are lives inside our vessel called a body. Who we are is ageless, timeless, ever-blossoming and evolving. Our bodies go through stages of growth and decay, leading to renewal of our physical forms and spiritual evolution.*

Stella was attending a spiritual retreat with her Grace community; some of her friends are 20-40 years younger than she. During some of the more physical activities, including nature walks and silent meditation walks, Stella felt the effects of her aging body: her hip was bothering her making the walking painful and difficult.

During the silent meditation Stella's thoughts turned to her noticing the details of her aging skin after her morning shower as she was applying lotion. Skin that once was supple, smooth and tight had become wrinkled, crinkled and loose. She sought clothing that would cover up the evidence, where once she felt free to bare her arms and legs. During her meditation as she was replaying her early-morning body scan, she felt tears falling down her cheeks, a lump in her throat, and the thought rushing through her mind shouting at her, "It's not fair! I don't feel old...and my body is slowly dying. I can see it!"

Stella was feeling sad. She was watching herself transition from the vibrant flower of youth to the withering leaf getting ready to replenish the soil as it falls to the ground. "I'm not ready to fall to the ground!" Stella was shouting to the Universe. "It's not fair…! I have more living to do!"

Stella's quiet little voice whispered: "Every stage of life is a miracle. Every stage of growth is beautiful." She felt her body tighten as she intentionally took a deep breath and leaned into her angry resistance to her body getting older.

Her teacher's words hit her in the heart: "Living your life from the place of soul can tell you many things that living your life from the place of mind and body alone cannot…"

Her husband's words hit her in her soul: *"What you see when you look at me is not me…what you feel in your heart is me…"*

Life was inviting Stella to focus on her soul essence, while accepting her aging body. Life was inviting Stella to step through her fear of aging and face the reality of living a *Big Love* life: loving herself for who she was.

12

Attachment

The more you tighten your grip, the more star systems will slip through your fingers. The most true thing I know about power: the more you clutch, the more you lose.

— Carrie Fisher

STELLA:	I can't let go of him!
ME:	What are you holding onto?
STELLA:	The way I feel with him when things are good?
ME:	And the times when things aren't good?
STELLA:	It's awful.
ME:	Tell me more…
STELLA:	I feel lonely, unseen, undervalued…
ME:	What is the percentage of times you feel wonderful versus awful?
STELLA:	10% wonderful — 90% awful.
ME:	Hmmm…

Stella is you…Stella is me. Stella was once addicted to Matt. She was once addicted to a specific feeling she craved. She was once addicted to a belief that was a Big Lie: she had believed that she could only have the feelings of passion with one specific lover despite his unavailability. She had also believed that Matt might change if she could hang onto their relationship long enough for him to wake up.

Then *she* woke up: she realized that she couldn't change anyone else; that her challenge was to accept herself and Matt, just as they both were, and to let go of insisting on anything. She let go of insisting that she could only have passion or happiness with one person. She let go of Matt. When she let go of him, she went through withdrawal, like any addiction. It took a long time. It wasn't easy. It was painful. And…it was liberating!

The Universe continued to send clients to Stella who were in addictive relationships. It was if she had been in training with her own life, so that she could assist others. Stella's client Jason sent a text, "I can't give up…I love her." Before Jason arrived for his next session, she reflected on her own struggle in letting go of Matt. It took Stella several years to let Matt go, which she finally did with love and gratitude, after over 30 breakups.

During that decade of her passionate dance with Matt, her coaches and friends offered well-meaning advice and guidance, wondering along with her what the payoff was for her. Stella was aware that Matt was sent to her as a gift so that she could learn on a deeper level about who she was and was not. Matt was her teacher and her lesson was self-love.

After their many years together, Stella sent Matt an email to say goodbye, because seeing him in person would have been too painful:

> *I will always love you and I'm grateful you've been in my life this past decade. I'm choosing to let you go because I don't miss how I feel when you cannot be available to me, when you cannot hold me close to your heart, when you are unable to allow yourself to love me as I love you. As we've discussed many times, I require reciprocity. I love*

you and I love me more. Thank you for all the experiences
of being alive we have shared. I wish you joy.

When Jason arrived for his session, Stella had just recalled her first kiss with Matt which took place in her office: Matt walked through her doorway like a proud warrior looking into her eyes as he approached her, kissing her... She noticed her heart sink when she saw Jason walk through her doorway; it wasn't Matt.

Stella brought herself back to center by approaching Jason with a long 20-second hug. She felt his sadness rush through her body. She quickly did some deep breathing as she prepared Jason's coffee, while she cleared his heavy energy from her system.

"I'm feeling your heavy heart, my dearest..." she observed as she handed Jason his cup of coffee. With tears welling up, he answered, "I just can't give up...I dream about Amy...I think about her all the time...it doesn't seem to matter how much she hurts and disappoints me!"

Stella explored with Jason what he believed about his one-sided relationship and his understanding of what Amy was capable of giving to him. He acknowledged that she wasn't capable of giving or loving the way he wanted. He believed that if he persisted his love would change her, somehow transform her into the perfect partner for him. He believed that he could never be sexually attracted to anyone else the way he was attracted to her.

"I'm wondering if you're willing to suspend some of your beliefs...what if your beliefs were not true? How would that change your choices?" She invited Jason to compare how he experienced himself with friends and family who value him and love him to how he feels with Amy. It was stunning to Stella to notice how Jason dismissed the love and dedication others showered upon him as he gripped his attachment to Amy.

Jason was defiant: "I can't let go of this deep belief that she needs me to show her love…that I can make a difference in her life, like no one else… "

Stella recognized Jason's obsession to prove something, like the Impossible-Dream syndrome. She was the last person to discourage anyone from having a big dream and pursuing a dream, despite impossible odds. In matters of the heart, she was aware that anything is possible. Her little voice whispered: "Ask him what he feels he needs to prove."

Stella looked at Jason, feeling her heart open with compassion for his deep pain: "What if love is more about letting go than holding on?"

"If I let go, it's like *giving up* on her…"

Stella took a deep breath and consulted Spirit for wisdom: "What if letting go is the ultimate statement about your love for yourself and your appreciation of everything of value you've experienced with Amy?"

Jason shouted: "I don't care about myself! I have to have her in my life!"

Stella held the silence and allowed the space for Jason to hear his own words… She then asked softly, "Is it true that you don't care about yourself…?" Jason started to sob. Stella held the space for him in her heart as she witnessed his pain and release.

As he quieted his sobs, wiping his face and sipping is coffee, he looked at Stella as if he just had some kind of epiphany: "It's not true…I just keep holding onto my attachment to Amy…believing I'll feel important and loved when she finally gives me what I want from her…"

60

Stella shared some love wisdom from Daniel Nielsen: "Fall in love with the soul first and intensify your lifetime love experience. It's really only when you are conscious of your soul that your ego-self submits and allows the heart to take control. That is true bliss, where the two merge and flow as one. Soul-deep loving. Real love."

Jason listened and sat in silence for several minutes. He then confessed, "I think my ego is getting in the way here, isn't it?"

Stella took his hand, gently squeezing it. "You're learning, my dearest. You're learning..."

13

Attraction

The people in my life are really mirrors of me.
This affords me the opportunity to grow and change.

— Louise Hay

STELLA:	Why am I attracting men who don't want commitment?
ME:	What you seek is seeking you.
STELLA:	I want a relationship.
ME:	Do you?
STELLA:	I'm not sure.
ME:	When you are clear and ready for commitment, the partner you are seeking will show up.

Stella is you…Stella is me. Stella wasn't sure. She didn't want to admit it but as much as she was longing for love and romance, she had to face that she was not ready for a long-term relationship. Her 32-year marriage was filled with turmoil and stress and she wanted peace and ease. The Universe continued to send her opportunities to get clear about who she was and what she wanted. Sometimes those opportunities were in the form of clients who were wrestling with similar issues. Sometimes the opportunities were meeting new men on her dating journey.

Richard showed up on her matches online. Stella reached out to him and after a couple of weeks, they arranged to meet for coffee. Their conversation was animated and deep. At one point, Richard looked over at Stella as if he was realizing something profound and declared, "I didn't expect to have this kind of conversation…" As they were saying goodbye, agreeing they would like to meet again, he looked at her almost wistfully saying, "I've got to think about this…"

After three phone conversations which were equally animated and transparent, each sharing much of substance, including Richard talking about his health concerns and Stella revealing her plans to move in with friends, Richard texted her "I don't think I'm ready to date…I'm going to step aside from that for now, and devote my efforts to music and politics…"

Stella knew when they met that while they had a satisfying intellectual connection, there was a lack of heart connection. She felt Richard's reserve. She had to admit she also felt some obstacles to her own heart opening to him. She pondered her connection with Richard. *I wonder if Richard was clear on what he was seeking. I also wonder about myself — do I believe that I can attract the person I really want to meet?*

14

What You Need

I love the idea that, as we look into someone's eyes, if we look long enough, we will see ourselves there. It is the "human gateway" into the experience of Oneness.

— Neale Donald Walsch

STELLA:	Why do I need him to love me?
ME:	Perhaps you believe that without his love, you aren't enough.
STELLA:	With his love, I imagine that I would feel complete...validated.
ME:	That word "validated" — such a sticky word isn't it?
STELLA:	Sticky?
ME:	Yes...in order for you to feel ok, you need someone else to "validate" that you're ok. Like validating your receipt at the restaurant for parking — they "validated" that you were in fact there.
STELLA:	Oh! Like I need "proof" that I'm really ok?
ME:	Exactly. So if he loves you, you've got the "proof" you need that "validates" your value, your worth, your merit...
STELLA:	That doesn't feel right...
ME:	Good. I think we're onto something.

Stella is you…Stella is me. In her younger years, Stella had been living with the illusion that if only the right people would love her, she would have the "proof" she thinks she needs to "validate" her worth. Without that proof, she didn't feel worthwhile or enough of whatever she believed she needed to feel good about herself.

Through her marriage, her professional life and extensive therapy, she began to understand that she was enough and that she was blessed to have Adam as her husband who loved her deeply, and to accept that other people in her life who did *not* love her was not about *her*. It was about *them*. That included her father and her stepchildren. She had learned to accept the reality that not everyone had the capacity to love her or anyone else; she learned that regardless of the capacity of others to love her, Stella would continue to be Stella.

Jason was due for another session, and she was looking for just the right words to share with him, since he was in deep pain and suffering over his feelings of love for a young woman who did not return to him the love and attention he craved. Without her love, he was convinced he was nothing. How could Stella get through to Jason? She found the words of Abraham:

> *"The Law of Attraction Assembles Happy Relationships… Asking your relationship with any other to be the basis of buoying you up is never a good idea, because the Law of Attraction cannot bring to you something different from the way you feel. The Law of Attraction cannot bring you a well-balanced, happy*

person if you are not yourself already that. The Law of Attraction, no matter what you do or say, will bring to you those who predominantly match the person who you predominantly are. Everything that everyone desires is for one reason only: they believe they will feel better in the having of it. We just want you to understand that you must feel better before it can come to you.

"In simple terms, if you are not happy with yourself, or with your life, the attraction of a partner will only exaggerate the discord, because any action taken from a place of lack is always counterproductive."

When Jason came into her office, she shared Abraham's wisdom. He had tears in his eyes as he said, "I keep thinking that I need her to love me before I can possibly feel better! This message is telling me that I must work to feel better about myself FIRST... How can I do that?"

Stella and Jason continued their conversation about what he believed about himself that created his obstacles to self-acceptance. Stella held Jason's heart gently in her own heart as they spoke. She intuitively *kythed* with Jason heart-to-heart, *"You are beautiful...you are enough,"* as she listened.

As Jason hugged Stella goodbye, he smiled and said: "I'm feeling calmer now...like you were doing magic of some kind."

Stella smiled: "Love is magic, isn't it?" Stella was feeling herself swimming in the sea of *Big Love*. It was delicious.

15

Blind Spots

We learn by reflecting on what we've done, where we've been, and what our relationships show us of ourselves.

— Sheila Pearl

STELLA: How do I know what my blind spots are?
ME: Whatever you don't like about your results
            is a clue.
STELLA: Like what?
ME: You say you want a life partner while you
            may not make time or space for one.
STELLA: Are you suggesting that perhaps I don't
            really want one?
ME: Maybe you're not ready to have one or
            maybe you're afraid of getting one?

Stella is you...Stella is me. She was not meeting "the One." Stella looked at her apartment and wondered: if she met a potential partner, would she want to invite him into her home? Would he have any place to put his stuff? She had been gradually creating a space which was anything *but* inviting to anyone – especially a potential partner. It was as if she was creating barriers and obstacles to finding "the One."

She felt a longing for sharing her life with one special person, yet her actions were saying the opposite: her living space was giving the opposite message. There was something deep inside of Stella that was holding up the "stop sign" for any movement in the direction of meeting "the One." What was that about?

She knew that it was inevitable that she would be leaving her home behind, moving out and into a house within a few months. She felt the sword of Damocles hanging over her head. What were Stella's blind spots?

The clues are in her results: a cluttered apartment, every closet full, every drawer full: no room for a partner. If Stella had believed she could meet "the One," she would have maintained her neat, elegant, and welcoming home. She would have allowed for space in her closets and drawers. Instead, every available space was taken, giving the energetic message: "no room here."

As Stella looked at her results, she wondered if she was somehow getting herself ready for her move: it was inevitable that she would be forced to vacate her home. It was too painful for her to face the realities of her choices and mistakes. She had become expert at finding ways to avoid facing her inevitable fate: she stayed away from home as much as possible. She was behaving like someone in mourning and didn't see it.

16

Feeling Homeless

Until you make the unconscious conscious,
it will direct your life and you will call it fate.

— Carl Jung

STELLA:	I'm feeling homeless.
ME:	Where is that feeling coming from?
STELLA:	I'm not sure.
ME:	Is "homeless" a place or a state of mind?
STELLA:	I'm guessing it's a state of mind.
ME:	So — describe your state of mind.
STELLA:	Empty. Cold. Disconnected. Lonely. Alone. Joyless.

Stella is you…Stella is me. Stella was feeling alone and disconnected. She felt a longing to experience connection and warmth, a sense of belonging and community. Since her mother passed, there was no longer any "home" for Stella to visit. Mama had always been home. Since Adam passed, she felt her own home was no longer home.

Gradually, year after year, Stella pulled away from doing the things she once did to create her home. Instead of inviting her friends to her home she visited friends in their homes, or they went out together. Instead of eating at home she often ate at the local diner, where people knew her and she felt at home. When she finally ended things with Matt she pulled further and further away from spending time in her own home.

Throughout her life with Adam, Stella had created a home environment that was colorful and elegant. She was proud of her beautiful china and dining room set. She took delight in having friends gather, spoiling them with a gourmet 4-course meal.

As the years passed after Adam's death, Stella hosted fewer dinner parties, often feeling a relief when she thought to herself, *Those are a thing of the past.* She had been slowly denying herself the experience of home: once a masterful cook, she seldom cooked. She was diminishing the importance of her home, minimizing the need for any of her belongings.

As Stella was anticipating her big move, she looked around her home and realized that her apartment had become simply a place to sleep at night, a place to store her belongings, and nothing much beyond that. She realized that she had been increasingly retreating *from* her residence, rather than retreating *to* her residence. Stella was pulling away from the connective tissue of everything that gave her the experience of "home."

As she was getting ready for her visit to California, her nostalgia continued to grab her heart: When her mother was alive, Stella was excited to go "home" to be with her mother. Theirs was a sweet and loving relationship. Stella had looked forward to cooking for her mother or working alongside one another in the kitchen preparing a festive meal for their family.

When Adam was alive, Stella was always enthusiastic about inviting friends and family for a meal and quality-time visits. She thrived in the midst of music playing in the background as friends and family engaged in lively conversation, laughter, and enjoyment of the meals she prepared.

As Stella sat in her bedroom, she asked herself, *How have I created this result?* She made an entry in her journal:

> *I'm grieving: I haven't yet allowed myself to fully grieve the loss of my life as it once was. Once I was a wife, mother, grandmother at the center of family gatherings in my home. Since Adam's illness, everyone stayed away. My home became an empty vessel. I began to feel like an empty vessel. Once I was a busy professional, a spiritual leader of my congregation. An educator in my Hebrew school. I was at the top of the mountain singing my song, teaching children and adults. At the center of the activities. Now, I'm alone in my coaching practice, never knowing who will come to me for my guidance, never knowing when I'm going to get the next phone call asking me to officiate at a wedding. I'm feeling more uncertainty and emptiness than ever before in my life. I feel like giving up. I feel like just walking away from my apartment...*

Stella could see that she needed help. She called her Grace friend to support her. Julie took Stella through the process of clarifying and releasing her resistance to her life circumstances, and her insistence on her situation being anything else, other than what it was. In the middle of their processing, Stella reminded herself of Stephen Levine's wisdom: "Hell is wishing that life be anything other than what it is."

Part of the process required Stella to be present to everything she was feeling. "Stay in that abyss...let yourself feel it." She had been resisting going there; didn't want to feel the deep sadness that was lurking in that dark deep place. Once Julie stayed with her, holding the space for her to feel everything, Stella allowed herself to cry, really cry. It was a deep cry that gave her the pathway to release her pain.

Julie waited for Stella to calm her tears. "How are you feeling now?"

Stella was feeling lighter and raw. "I'm feeling alive again. When I got to that *whatever* place, it felt like death. Thank you my beloved! I'm awake now."

17

Mysteries & Miracles

*Faith and fear both demand you believe in something
you cannot see. You choose.*

— Bob Proctor

STELLA: Yesterday I couldn't imagine HOW I could
           gather enough cash together to buy a
           round-trip ticket to California, and today
           the money showed up!

ME: It sounds like miracles are happening all
           around you...

STELLA: I can't believe I'm going home to finally see
           family and friends *plus* meet Wally in
           person!

ME: Interesting — you didn't want a long-
           distance relationship.

STELLA: Yes...it was Wally who said to me,
           "Distance is but an illusion."

ME: Yet...you're leaning into the distance issue
           and meeting him in your hometown. It
           seems like an unusual opportunity...

Stella is you...Stella is me. Stella had co-created a sweet long-distance friendship with Wally who lives 1000 miles away. They agreed to be friends without any focus on future, proximity, or distance. Through phone calls and online connection, they had established a heart-centered friendship.

Wally called Stella and offered her an unusual opportunity: to visit California when he was there for a conference. He would be speaking near Stella's hometown, where she was born and had family and friends. She knew she could stay with her lifelong friend Shirley, and Wally was inviting her as his guest at the B&B near the conference. Stella didn't know how she would raise the money for the airfare, yet she trusted it would happen. Wally and Stella had established a ritual together in which they set an intention for something and trusted that Spirit would provide.

Just as Stella was planning to call her friend Shirley to ask if she could stay during her visit, Shirley called Stella to let her know if she wanted to stay one more time in Shirley's home, it would have to be soon. Shirley and her husband were packing up to move. Stella had already listened to her little voice, "Go! Now is the time!" She didn't have money in her account on Monday. Tuesday was the deadline for making her flight plans at the lowest possible fare. On Tuesday morning, she received payments from her clients which provided the funds Stella needed.

"I got my ticket!" she squealed to Wally during their phone call.

"Oh sweetheart! That's so beautiful! We will have a wonderful visit! I can't wait to introduce you to my friends!" Wally was excited about sharing meals and conversation with Stella…in person.

Stella couldn't wait to hug him. She was also excited to see her dear friends and family.

18

What Is Home?

Only those who care about you can hear you when
you are quiet.

— Robert Stack

STELLA: I just got my ticket…I'm **so** excited!
ME: Where are you going?
STELLA: Home.
ME: Where's home?

Stella is you…Stella is me. Stella was feeling the clock ticking. It had been three years since she visited her childhood friend and family in her hometown. She suddenly had an opportunity to finally meet Wally. For her, meeting him would be a dream come true. She often felt an impulse to hug him during their many phone conversations.

Since she had connected with Wally, Stella had a strange sense that he was "home" for her. She had begun to realize that "home" was less about a place and more about where her heart was connected. Her trip would be a homecoming for her in many ways.

Stella flew into Long Beach which was easier for Shirley to navigate. Once Stella got her luggage, she texted Shirley "I'm here. I'll meet you at the curb outside baggage claim."

It had been three years since she had visited with Shirley, yet when Stella saw her dear friend, it was if they had seen each other the day before.

"Your hair is pure white!" Stella shouted. Shirley had stopped dying her hair dark brown, and for Stella it was a shock to see her friend with all-white hair. They hugged and giggled as they both looked at each other, assessing how each other looked.

"You look just the same, Stella!" Shirley smiled.

Stella laughed: "Ha! — Yes, I just have to work harder to create the illusion that I've got hair!"

When they arrived at Shirley's home, Stella felt a familiar nostalgia: this was the house she had been visiting for nearly 45 years. Shirley helped Stella take her bags up the stairs to the guest room Stella had been enjoying all those years.

Stella looked around: "I'm taking it all in…I know you won't be in this house when I visit you next…" Stella looked around Shirley's home and could see how Shirley and her husband were already purging their belongings, getting ready for their move. Stella felt a sadness: Shirley's house had become "home" for Stella when she visited friends and family in her hometown.

19

My Mirrors

Treat everyone as if you're looking in the mirror —
because you are.

— Sheila Pearl

STELLA:	He called me "sweetheart" before we met, and now…nothing.
ME:	Sounds like something changed.
STELLA:	Once we met in person, the energy shifted.
ME:	What changed?
STELLA:	I sensed he wasn't interested in me at all…

Stella is you…Stella is me. Stella finally met Wally. True: they had agreed to be purely "Agape" friends yet had established a sweet loving connection before meeting in person. They called one another "sweetheart" and "honey" during their phone conversations. They looked forward to meeting at the conference where they would be able to spend quality time getting to know one another better.

Stella arrived at the conference venue and Wally greeted her with a hug and kiss. It was warm and affectionate. She was looking forward to deepening their friendship during the following few days.

However, after a few hours of her arrival and their initial greeting, she noticed a strange shift. After an early evening of dinner with friends, they had the time to relax in Stella's room, to engage in conversation, but Wally declined the option. Stella was incredulous that Wally was disinterested in grabbing the rare opportunity to dig deeper in getting to know one another. After all, the evening was still young. It was only 8:00pm! She went to her room and relaxed before retiring, feeling dismissed and ignored by a man who had expressed a desire to connect and discover each other.

The day Stella was returning to Shirley's house, Wally joined her for coffee. Still feeling confused by his dismissal of her two nights prior, she observed something she hadn't realized until that moment: Wally never asked about her. Every part of the conversation centered on him. She was trying mightily not to take this personally, but it was true: Wally wasn't curious about her. He just wasn't interested. She wondered what she might have done or said that changed the energy between them.

Stella reflected on her role in their friendship: she was the listener. She was there to be his audience. There was little reciprocity. For her, without reciprocity, there was no divine flow of energy. He did not seem interested in Stella. His only interest was in her being attentive to him. She felt lonely with him. When she returned to Shirley's home, Stella felt seen and heard. There, she was "home" with her dear friend.

Stella's first client after returning to New York from her trip, Ella, had just made a discovery about a man she had dated a few times: "He didn't seem interested in me and my pleasure...it was as if I was there to serve his needs, and I felt invisible and irrelevant".

Stella understood, as she reflected on her own recent disappointment. "Either a person understands their own power to transform a partner by paying close attention to their partner, or they live forever as a selfish adolescent who acts as if it's all about them and their own needs. When a person awakens to their role as lover, they open the doorway to bliss."

Ella nodded her head. She knew that she wanted a lover — an awakened man whose deepest pleasure was his knowing he had pleased her by being fully present to her. Stella reminded Ella that there were awakened men out there.

"Why is it so difficult to meet the man for me?!?" cried Ella.

"Embrace the process. With each person you meet, you learn more about yourself. It's all a part of your own growth. Lighten up. He will show up."

When Ella came for her next session with Stella, she almost skipped into the room. "This guy just fell out of the sky! I've already met him twice this week. He's that awakened man you've been talking about. I feel so at home with him! He wants to know me. He's curious. He pays attention!"

Stella smiled as Ella reflected on this new man who had magically appeared. He had found Ella online. He pursued her. He initiated their phone conversation. He invited her for lunch and chose the restaurant after asking what kind of food she liked. Ella was experiencing the benefits of being in the company of an awakened man: he was primarily interested in her. He didn't make the conversation about himself. Their conversation was reciprocal. There was the divine flow of energy going on. Ella wasn't feeling lonely: she was feeling included and seen.

Stella felt a twinge of sadness, even slight jealousy as she witnessed the miracle of Ella meeting the partner she had envisioned possible for her. Stella was happy for Ella, at the same time she felt that deep longing to feel included and seen by a loving partner.

As above, so below... Stella reminded herself. She remained determined to envision what she believed to be possible for herself, even though it was not yet in front of her face.

20

Empathy

*Love opens us up to all that life has to offer. But first,
we must learn to love ourselves with all our flaws
and imperfection…when you love yourself, you set
yourself free to receive love and to give love away to
others.*

— Daniel Nielsen

STELLA: It wasn't about me…

ME: What wasn't about you?

STELLA: His preoccupation with himself…

ME: Of course — it was never about you!

STELLA: I'm not taking it personally that he was self-absorbed.

ME: That's very good news.

STELLA: I was taking it personally and now I'm not.

ME: How does that change things for you?

STELLA: Now I can feel empathy for him.

Stella is you…Stella is me. Stella was disappointed about her visit with Wally. He seemed preoccupied and self-absorbed throughout their visit; she took it personally that Wally was distracted and didn't pay attention to her. He did not seem to be himself, or the Wally she had grown to know and love before they met in person.

After they had both returned to their homes after the California visit, Wally wrote to Stella, apologizing: "Forgive me for not being myself. I had a scare with my blood pressure and was feeling terrified about my health throughout my trip to California. When I returned home, I went to the emergency room when I had another dizzy spell like I had in California after I first arrived. The doctors told me that I was at great risk. I know I didn't pay attention to you because I was so derailed by my fear."

Stella felt a surge of shame rush through her body as she read Wally's email. *I was making it all about me, when it wasn't at all. What I was thinking!*

Stella called Wally to inquire about his health. "I'm much better now. I just feel terrible that we couldn't have the quality visit I had hoped for…"

Stella understood. "I'm just sorry you couldn't let me know what was going on with you. You didn't have to keep it to yourself…don't you know I'm the first person who would understand?"

Wally and Stella pledged to remain soul friends and to accept the limitations of living 1000 miles apart. Wally reminded Stella of his promise: "I will always love you, in a very big way. A *Big Love* way. Let's remind ourselves of the beauty of our soul connection. Let it be what it is."

Stella realized that she was looking at the very big opportunity of loving Wally on a soul level, without expectations of anything at all, except their loving heart connection. She smiled at herself. "Am I making our soul connection something *less* than a romantic connection? Isn't it really *Big Love* that I have been craving all along? Don't I already have what it is I want?"

Stella *kythed* with Wally: *"You are love, joy, and courage."* She enjoyed her soul connection with him.

As she was in her meditative state, connecting with him, she received a message: *"You are beautiful and delicious..."* Was this an intuitive message from Wally? Did it matter who sent it? What mattered was that Stella believed it. She continued to maintain her connection with Wally. Another message came to her: *"He is a reflection of your own fears and fragility about you life at this stage of your life. When you can accept your own fear and feelings of fragility, you can more deeply empathize with his."*

Stella smiled to herself as she felt a deep gratitude for her soul connection. She was feeling her heart expand: it was *Big Love*.

21

Seeing Me

Light must come from inside. You cannot ask the
darkness to leave;
you must turn on the light.

— Sogyal Rinpoche

STELLA:	I miss the way he looked at me…
ME:	Tell me how you felt about yourself when he looked at you?
STELLA:	Like I was the only person he could see at that moment…
ME:	What else?
STELLA:	Like I mattered to him…
ME:	What else?
STELLA:	Like he saw me, really saw me…
ME:	Was there anyone else who also gave you that experience of yourself?
STELLA:	Yes. Mama.

Stella is you…Stella is me. Stella maintained her friendship with Wally and their connection filled her heart with joy. Nonetheless, in the silence and solitude she experienced when she was home, facing the inevitable move out of the apartment which had been her home for 16 years, out of the space she had last shared with Adam before his death, she felt Adam's presence all around her. She often missed Adam so deeply, she broke out in sobs, sometimes just quiet tears gently falling down her face.

She often missed Adam most when she was with someone who didn't see her or didn't seem to want to know her, really know her. She also missed her mother, who had been her best friend and confidant for a lifetime. Stella missed the connection. She missed the feeling she experienced when someone she loved looked into her eyes and felt seen...really seen. Stella knew her value; she loved herself. It was an ongoing process, nonetheless: she missed Adam and her Mama who had been clarifying mirrors for her: she loved what she saw in their eyes.

Stella's reverie was interrupted by Jason's text: "I'm struggling...do you have time today?"

Jason was struggling with his self-esteem and admitted to Stella that he didn't understand what self-love was about. He believed that he would grow to love himself when the "right person" loved him. His challenge was twofold: first, the young woman he wanted to love him was not emotionally available to him, except occasionally as "just a friend." Second, he was placing his own emotional stability and love for himself in the hands of someone else.

Stella asked Jason about where he was emotionally.

"I just want her to look at me all the time the way she did that one night on the lake...why can't she just pay attention to me that way every time I see her?!"

Stella felt Jason's pain. When Amy had looked deeply into his eyes that one time during a heartfelt conversation, Jason experienced being seen by her. He felt the close connection with her, and in that one conversation, he believed she wanted to know more about him. He wanted to know about her. There was what Stella often described as "the divine flow of energy" in which both people were engaged in a sweet connection of reciprocity. Stella often made reference to her own experience of that "divine flow of energy" with her husband. She understood Jason's deep longing to experience that connection on a consistent basis.

Jason's choice of partner became his most important mirror — painful and instructive. Amy was not emotionally capable of being consistent about anything, especially her relationships. She was very young and emotionally immature. Jason was ten years her senior, and for people in their 20s and 30s, that was a big difference.

"When else have you felt the way you felt that night?" Stella inquired.

"Never…"

Stella understood that Jason needed to appreciate the people in his life who did love and value him; she knew that Jason's grandmother treated Jason as if he was the center of her Universe, and that he had a few good friends who had his back. "When you're with your grandmother or your good friend Ken, how would you describe your connection?"

Jason began to realize that other friends gave him the experience of being seen, heard and appreciated.

"I suggest you spend more quality time with your friends and family who love you and appreciate you, and less time chasing Amy."

Jason confessed that Amy had become the "impossible dream" for him, almost as if he had to "prove" something to himself.

Stella reminded Jason: "Love is not something you have to prove, like winning a contest. It's something you are, and you give it away. The kind of love you are seeking is *Big Love*. It starts with loving yourself in a very big way."

Stella reflected on her own experiences of the "divine flow of energy" and reminded herself of the very few times she felt that with Matt. She wanted it to be consistent, and Matt could not sustain it. She took it personally, instead of seeing Matt as a gift — someone who, on a soul level, was showing Stella who she was. It was Stella's job to receive the gift and integrate the experience on a soul level, accepting that magic that happens once can become an eternal moment.

Stella looked at Jason with great compassion; she understood his struggle: "Amy gave you a gift that night at a lake...she was your mirror, showing you to yourself, so you could remember how beautiful and magnificent you are."

Jason couldn't hold back the tears. He felt the truth of what Stella was showing him. "I will try to remember..."

Stella understood that Jason was learning...still learning.

After Jason left her office, Stella had an hour before her next client. She decided to meditate on the question *When do I feel seen?* She recorded her answers in her journal:

> *I feel seen by my good friends Cat and Donna; by my Goddesses on Monday nights, by my dear friend Orah, by many of my clients in the midst of our most intimate conversations, by my Grace community brothers and sisters, and by my lifetime friends Shirley and Rae.*

> *I feel seen when I'm in the midst of my own vulnerability and authenticity with others, whether it's my friends, family or clients; I also feel seen when I'm deeply involved in my authentic passion in my work, whether it's while I'm singing or speaking.*

22

Divine Flow

I believe in everything until it's disproved. So I
believe in fairies, the myths, dragons. It all exists,
even if it's in your mind. Who's to say that dreams
and nightmares aren't as real as the here and now?

— John Lennon

STELLA:	Can I trust this amazing feeling of oneness?
ME:	Tell me more.
STELLA:	Everything about us just flows…
ME:	Everything?
STELLA:	Our conversation, our loving interaction.
ME:	Tell me more about your question.
STELLA:	It all feels too good to be true…I'm almost afraid to trust it.
ME:	Oh! You're having doubts about what you've manifested?

Stella is you…Stella is me. Stella was reflecting on Jason and Wally. She felt deep empathy for Jason's struggle and his desire to feel *oneness* with that one special person. She understood his hunger to *be in love.* Like Jason, she wanted to feel the bliss of *oneness* again.

Like Jason, Stella appreciated her friends especially friends like Wally. She enjoyed their soul connection, and they often experienced oneness in their connection. Nonetheless, like Jason, she was craving the bliss that comes from the combination of erotic love with the biggest love, called Agape. She wasn't sure it was something she would ever experience again.

Stella reflected back 45 years on the magic of meeting Adam.

Her roommate had invited her to meet friends of hers for cocktails and dinner. Stella was 29, an aspiring opera singer. As she approached the lounge where she was meeting Diane, she felt someone looking at her. It was Adam who was sitting next to Diane.

Before Stella reached their table, Adam leaned over to Diane and said, "That blonde who is walking over here will be my wife someday…"

Diane laughed, saying, "You're crazy! That's my roommate Stella who is joining us tonight."

Adam smiled as he fixed his gaze on Stella: "That will make it easier."

Stella had suffered several disappointments and losses before she met Adam that night. She was afraid to trust and kept Adam at arms' length for weeks. Adam had a deep intuitive *knowing* that Stella was destined to be his life partner. He pursued her relentlessly, and eventually won her heart.

Stella struggled with her doubts: she couldn't fathom to experience the kind of *oneness* she had enjoyed with Adam again.

She believed that the Universe had reserved only one such experience for her. She forgot that she had everything to say about what the Universe had provided for her. She had the illusion that her experience of *oneness* depended on one specific magical romantic relationship. She was sucked in by the Big Lie; she was challenged to acknowledge the truth about life. When she opened her heart and mind to possibilities, she could imagine what *Big Love* could be for herself and others.

Stella was holding her *kything* workshop. She always began with a gentle chant she had composed: *"Listen to your Heartsong"* and told the story of her first *kything* experience with Adam, when he was in the final stages of his dementia:

> *"I walked into Adam's room when he was asleep, sat on the sofa and began the* kything *process. I closed my eyes, began my deep breathing, had a clear intention of dropping down from my head to my heart. From that heart center, I imagined a beautiful gold cord extending from my heart to his. I then silently intuitively repeated my* kythe: 'I love you…I miss you…I miss hearing your voice.'

> *"Within a few minutes, I heard his voice say:* 'I've been waiting for you to find a way to hear my voice…. What you see when you look at me is not me. What you feel with your heart is me. Keep listening.'"

Stella continued explaining the primary benefit of the experience of *kything*: "Oneness is a knowing that we are not separate from Source...and that we are interconnected with one another."

Stella felt a warmth wash over her, like sweet kisses and gentle hugs. Often when she was preparing for her *kything* workshops, or officiating at a wedding, she would feel that warmth all around and through her body. She recognized it as a sweet combination of her daughter Daedra's, her mother's, and Adam's essence each whispering through her heart, *"I'm here...I'm always here."*

Ella was due for her appointment at 4:30. At 2:30, Stella received a confirmation text message from Ella with a link to Rachmaninoff's Rhapsody — one of Stella's favorites. "I'm thinking of you. See you at 4:30." How did Ella know that *that* piece of music was especially meaningful to Stella? How did she choose the exact piece of music that Stella played at night to lull Daedra to sleep? This was *oneness*.

Stella often heard Daedra's spirit whispering in her ear, *"I'm with you mama...I'm sending you children all the time. Know that I'm always with you."* She felt that warm hug, like her mother's loving hand on her shoulder. That feeling of being cherished like Adam's kiss on her forehead. That experience of tenderness like Matt's nuzzling and nibble kisses. Stella reminded herself, *These are the eternal moments that remind me who I am.*

Ella arrived at exactly 4:30. She walked in Stella's office with a calm grace. She wasn't giddy. She was in a state of peace and ease. "I can't explain it...when we're together, I have such a feeling of oneness. For the first time in my life, I'm not wondering where this is going. I know where we are. I'm at peace being present. I know we are one."

As Stella listened to Ella, she recognized herself.

23

Clarity

Live life as if everything has been rigged in your favor.

— Rumi

STELLA:	I want what she has!
ME:	Sounds like you're jealous…
STELLA:	No. I'm clear.
ME:	Sounds like you are coming from a mindset of lacking something someone else has…
STELLA:	Until she got what she has now she had a clear vision about what she wanted, and she kept going until she reached her goal.
ME:	So, you see her as a role model for getting what you want?
STELLA:	Yes. I'm not settling for less.

Stella is you…Stella is me. Stella was longing for a close loving relationship. She was frustrated by the dating process and often felt like giving up. She was wrestling with her inner voices: "You already have what you want, you already have within you everything you need. Pay attention to what is right in front of your face!"

Ella arrived for her session early and Stella felt a giddiness in Ella's energy. "You have that look on your face that says you have something wonderful to tell me."

Ella covered her face with her hands as she giggled and blushed. "We spent the whole weekend together. It was magical. I didn't want to leave..." Stella knew. This was the one for Ella. "I feel like a princess and I'm living a dream!"

Stella thought about her date with Jim the night before and felt a twinge of jealousy as Ella embellished on her magical weekend of loving connection with her new boyfriend. "I can't believe this is happening! He's everything I've ever wanted! He's everything I put on my list two years ago. I'm so grateful for all those guys who disappointed me! They brought me to Don!"

Stella received a text from Jim in the midst of Ella's report of her weekend activities. "What do you say? Dinner Wednesday?" Stella wasn't interested. She had no desire to see Jim. She mused to herself as Ella was sharing her magical weekend news: "I want what she has..."

In the past, Stella had coached Ella through her many dark nights of the soul, through painful disappointments, rejections, and feelings of despair in ever meeting the right partner for her. "Hold the space for the fact that whatever you are seeking is seeking you." Ella had nodded and smiled as she wrote that in her journal: *what you seek is seeking you.*

Now, the poet Rumi was in the room, reminding Stella of the wisdom she had shared with Ella long ago. After Ella's session, Stella picked up her own journal and turned to her January 1st entry:

> *My life partner has a very big heart. It is a generous open heart. He is confident in himself, accepts, loves, and honors himself.*

My partner is abundant in every way. His financial abundance is a reflection of his spiritual awareness. He loves his work and is passionate about his life.

My partner is healthy. In body. In emotions. In spirit. He takes good care of all aspects of his well-being.

My partner loves many kinds of music, including the classics. He loves to learn new things, including cooking and food. He loves to travel and loves staying home as well.

My partner loves to kiss, cuddle, and make love in a variety of ways. He is a lover. He is a giver. He is a nurturer.

Stella looked at her entry, and realized it was a mirror of herself, except for one aspect: financial abundance actually showing up in her bank account. She wondered if this was the one aspect of herself which she needed to allow to flourish. She believed that she was and had always been abundant. *I want to be in alignment with myself.* She then thought about Jim and asked herself, *Is this who Jim is? Is this who I am?* The answer is, *No.*

She then responded to Jim's text about dinner that week: "I'm not going to continue seeing you. The energy isn't a good fit for me. I wish you well."

Stella reflected on her longings. She realized that what Ella was experiencing was what Stella had once lived: a dream come true. Stella wrestled with the real and the fantasy in her life: she had a fantastical — almost unbelievable — life at one time, which then became a nightmare and transformation through painful challenges with their loving connection. Stella's current challenge was to get real with herself about what *she* wanted at this time in her life. Stella wasn't Ella.

24

Dying

Be like a tree and let the dead leaves drop.

— Rumi

STELLA:	I'm afraid to die now!
ME:	What's your fear?
STELLA:	Not living my dream...
ME:	So, dying isn't your fear?
STELLA:	No. It's about time.
ME:	What if time is an illusion?
STELLA:	I need more time to complete my work.
ME:	So you think...

Stella is you...Stella is me. Stella received a call from her brother. It was about her nephew, Jake. His heart condition was serious; he needed a new heart. He couldn't wait. He had to have a pump installed in his chest to keep his heart pumping while he waited for a new heart. The surgery was risky. There were no guarantees. Stella felt a cold sweat rush through her body as her brother described the grave situation.

Stella reflected on her diagnosis of cancer when she was 45.

The doctors gave her the worst-case scenario. The cold-sweat of terror rushed throughout her body. She imagined going through chemo, her hair falling out, and at the end of the process dying before her time anyway. She shouted to the moon, to the Universe, "I'm not ready to die yet!"

She had six weeks between her first and second surgery. She gathered data, resources, did research on alternative approaches to self-healing, and compiled a list of what she required at Sloan-Kettering before and after her second surgery. During her six weeks, she meditated daily and played healing music as she envisioned her body clean of the cancer. She boosted her immune system with supplements and foods rich in phytonutrients.

Stella instructed her medical team to give her intravenous vitamin C and B12 before and after surgery. At first they refused, but Stella threatened to go home unless they agreed. The night before surgery she settled into her bed at the hospital and meditated one last time as she played soothing music and envisioned her body being free and clear of the cancer which her doctors told her had most likely metastasized throughout her lymphatic system. She envisioned her body being clean.

Four days after Stella's surgery, her medical team came to her bedside. The surgeon smiled as he scratched his ear: "Stella...we don't quite know how to explain this...but we found nothing. You are completely clean..."

Stella started to cry as Adam grabbed her hand. "Oh, my God! I'm not surprised...I'm just grateful!"

The team attempted to convince Stella and Adam that chemo and radiation were recommended as preventive measures. Stella refused the chemo. Adam pressured her to agree to radiation.

Four weeks after her second surgery, Stella auditioned for her dream job. She got the job! She became the Cantor for a large congregation in New Jersey. As she was preparing the music for the holidays, she was also undergoing the radiation treatments. Amidst nausea and weakness, Stella's passion for her work gave her the energy to move forward.

I knew I wasn't ready to die yet! I knew something was ahead of me...

Stella was gathering positive energy for her call to her nephew Jake before his surgery. She wanted to be a voice of courage and strength for him; she didn't want him to hear any fear in her voice. Then the night before his surgery came — she couldn't wait any longer. She took a deep breath and decided to *kythe* with him first: "You are love...you are joy...you are courage."

When Jake answered the phone, he reassured Stella: "I know I'll be ok...I have a strong feeling that everything will go well." He sounded so sure. He had a quiet knowing.

She recognized that knowing. She mirrored his faith: "I'm trusting that the Universe has your back and your medical team does too...we are all praying for you, my darling!"

Stella ended the call and broke into sobs. She was struggling with her fears for her precious nephew. He had always been like a son to her. He was only 46 — about the same age she was 30 years earlier when she faced death — and had been fighting for his life throughout a harrowing struggle.

Finally, his medical team decided he would be a candidate for a heart transplant. His heart was failing, and he couldn't wait for a heart to become available. An LVAD pump was installed in his body to keep his heart pumping while he awaited a new heart. It was all risky. During the previous two years, Jake had been on the edge of death several times — the LVAD pump was his last chance to buy time, while they waited for a new heart.

Stella watched the clock: his surgery was at 8:00am. It was noon. She waited to hear from her brother. Hours went by. Stella couldn't work. She was frozen in fear. "Trust in the Universe..." She kept repeating to herself. "He somehow knows he'll be okay...just trust..."

Stella had learned to let go of attachment to the outcome. This was her nephew. It was almost impossible to let go... She wrestled with her fear. The cold sweat kept rushing through her body. She kept breathing. *Kything*. Praying. Breathing. *Kything*. Praying.

At 3:00pm, she got a text from her brother: "He's out of surgery. Doc says it went very well!"

Her brother's text was like music to her ears. She continued to *kythe* with Jake, "*You are love...you are joy...you are courage.*"

25

Feeling Everything

The wound is the place where light enters you.

— Rumi

STELLA:	I just want to live a happy life and feel none of that negative stuff.
ME:	So…you want only sunshine, and no rain?
STELLA:	Right.
ME:	So…you want only smiles, and no tears?
STELLA:	Right.
ME:	It seems you want to live in la-la land and not in real life…
STELLA:	What's wrong with that?!?
ME:	The law of opposites is just as real a law in life as gravity. There is no up without down. There is no joy without sorrow. There is no light without darkness.

Stella is you…Stella is me. Stella was experiencing the "law of opposites" more every day as she got clearer and more awake about herself and her life circumstances. She sometimes just wanted to fall asleep and stay numb to her feelings. It sometimes seemed like it would be so much easier. The more Stella's life circumstances became overwhelming, the more she had the impulse to escape those feelings of fear and anxiety. Her clients often became her best teachers and kept her awake, even though she wanted to sleep.

Stella's client Wanda had just celebrated four years of sobriety. Friends and family were congratulating her, some sending cards and flowers. Wanda told Stella she was disappointed her boyfriend didn't send flowers. "Let's go back to my first rule for loving connections: expect zero. It helps so you don't set yourself up for disappointment."

Wanda seemed poised for battle as she took a deep breath: "Don't you think he should have made it a big deal?!"

Stella reminded Wanda of the various ways her addiction had left its mark: "It seems you look for ways to be wronged or disappointed, almost as if those are comfortable places for you to be…"

Wanda's dark eyes glistened. "I just want him to give me those good feelings!"

Stella asked Wanda a question she asked often: "Can anyone else give you the feelings you have?"

Stella and Wanda explored those darker emotions which had kept her a prisoner of alcohol and substance abuse for decades. Stella summed up their discussion: "You were addicted to those substances most of your adult life because you could not tolerate the darker, negative emotions which are inevitable in life. You would seek ways to numb and float in your artificial nirvana."

Wanda nodded her head in agreement. "So now that I'm awake, my greatest challenge is to be willing to feel disappointed and vulnerable!"

Stella nodded her head with a smile. "Yes — that's the price of being aware, awake, and sober."

26

Blessings in Disguise

*The most authentic thing about us is our capacity to
create, to overcome, to endure, to transform, to love,
and...to be greater than our suffering.*

– Ben Okr

STELLA:	Why did my child die?
ME:	Ask a different kind of question.
STELLA:	What are you talking about?!?!
ME:	Your questions will define your quality of life...
STELLA:	What's missing in my question?
ME:	The assumption that the Universe has your back.
STELLA:	How can my child's death be a blessing?

Stella is you...Stella is me. Stella was in an extremely vulnerable place: she was observing the anniversary (*yahrzeit*) of her daughter's and stepdaughter's death. The anniversary dates were one day apart, making March 6-7 a time of sacred reflection and honoring of memory. Her stepdaughter died at 55 after a long illness. As Stella stood by her grandchildren's side at the funeral, it was surreal and familiar.

For over 50 years, Stella had mourned the death of her infant daughter. In her youth, Stella kept asking, "Why me?" "Why her?"

She kept feeling like a victim of circumstances, seeing life through the lens of "Life is happening TO me!"

Decades later, Stella's teacher suggested she ask a different kind of question: "How can I make this tragedy a blessing?" That was the question Stella was asking herself at her stepdaughter's funeral. She was focused on being there for her grandchildren who had lost their mother. In her daily work, Stella was dedicated to supporting men and women who were wrestling with the tough issues of life, especially loss and bereavement.

Stella got a call from Gail, a referral from a colleague. "My therapist thinks I need your wisdom. I hate myself and need your help."

Gail had two teenage daughters who were angry and defiant. Gail's husband was giving up on their marriage, saying, "I'm exhausted trying to fix you..." Stella didn't want to step into the same trap. She didn't want to fix Gail. She wanted to remind Gail of who she had always been and forgot.

"How can you make all your childhood abuse and your own substance abuse a blessing to you and your family now?"

Gail looked at Stella with tears welling up as she fought to push down that lump in her throat. "How can any of that nightmare be a blessing?!?!" Gail's eyes were on fire with defiance.

"What if everything that happens in our lives is **for** us and we have the opportunity to turn it into a gift of learning and growing in specific ways?"

Gail looked down as she confessed, "I'm treating my daughters the way I was treated...and they hate me..."

Stella asked Gail what the truth was about her relationship with her girls.

"If I don't care about them, they can't hurt me…"

Stella explored what Gail believed versus what was true.

"Okay, okay! What's true is I'm afraid of caring about my daughters… what's also true is that I love my daughters, but don't want them to know I care…"

Stella observed, "So…it seems that what's true is that you're afraid of being vulnerable…"

Gail admitted, "Of course! I've created a strong defense to protect myself from being hurt!"

"Hmm…it seems that the more you guard against being hurt, you create distance between you and the people in your life who really matter to you…"

Gail asked, "How can I keep my heart open?"

"Stay present to what is true. What you've just told me is that it's true you love your daughters. Be authentic about what's true…." Stella reminded her.

Gail looked at Stella as if she just had some kind of epiphany. "I wish you had been my mother…"

Stella felt a familiar lump in her throat. "I wish I had been your mother too…and I'm here now."

27

Depression

The depression belongs to all of us.

I think of the family down the road whose mother was having a baby and they went around the neighborhood saying, "We're pregnant." I want to go around the neighborhood saying, "We're depressed." If my mum can't get out of bed in the morning, all of us feel the same. Her silence has become ours, and it's eating us alive!

— Batish

STELLA:	My husband's depression was my depression.
ME:	How did you protect yourself?
STELLA:	It was like breathing secondary smoke.
ME:	There was no escape?
STELLA:	When a smoker blows the smoke in your face, how do you escape the smoke?
ME:	Surely there is a way to remain unaffected…

Stella is you…Stella is me. Stella recognized that she was suffering from depression. She had reached out for help from her coaches and spiritual community.

While married to Adam, Stella often battled depression. Her mother understood. Sometimes Stella was convinced that her mother was a witch, because she always seemed to know when to call to check up on Stella.

"So...what are you wearing right now?" her Mama would ask.

Often Stella would have to confess she was wearing her nightgown, although it was the middle of the afternoon.

"Take a shower, make your bed, get dressed, and go take a walk." This was Mama's reminder that Stella needed to change her energy, stay in motion, and go out to meet her world.

Stella, already prone to depression herself, was married to a man who was depressed, fearful, and angry. Adam was also a brilliant and funny man. She had seen brilliant and funny when she married him; but she didn't see the depth of his depression until later.

Several months before they were to be married, Adam's eldest son was tragically killed in a car accident. The effect of that loss was a permanent wound for everyone in the family. Adam's other two children came to live with Stella and Adam after their marriage. The entire family was depressed, fearful and angry.

That was the emotional backdrop that surrounded Stella in her home. It was the underpinnings of the household's energy.

Decades later in their marriage, when Adam developed dementia, his disease became Stella's daily reality — just like living in a household of depressed people.

Stella's challenge for three decades had been to navigate her daily life with positivity, in the midst of the negativity. How did she create the positivity?

I immerse myself in my passion. Stella's daily antidote to living in a sea of negativity was love: her passion for her work. She had always been a singer. She found a way to leverage her skills and talents to serve a congregation as a Cantor and spiritual leader. It was her love for music and people that created a kind of energetic shield that protected her immune system.

Wanda walked into Stella's office with a heaviness in her step; her face looked ashen and lifeless. "I can't take it anymore! My heart is breaking, and I don't know how to escape the heaviness of depression in my household!"

Wanda's partner was depressed, her son and daughter were depressed, and Wanda was in recovery from addiction — fighting a daily battle to overcome her own demons while feeling the effects of the epidemic of depression all around her. "How can I protect myself from this pervasive poison?!" she shouted.

"What are you passionate about?"

Wanda sat motionless for a few seconds, then whispered, "Dancing! I'm passionate about my music and feeling joy when I dance." Stella silently held the space for Wanda to recognize her passions. "I also love my work. I love to help others. I'm passionate about helping others to overcome their addictions."

Stella and Wanda discussed how they each had been living the truth that taught, "We are in this together".

There is no escape. *Big Love* is the antidote.

28

It Is Hopeless

*When you bear witness to your responses to life's
current events and immediately retract what you
decided in the past about similar events, you give
yourself almost unimaginable power — including the
power to end struggle and suffering forever. Buddha
demonstrated this precisely, and taught it.*

— Neale Donald Walsch

STELLA: I'm feeling it's all so hopeless…

ME: I'm hearing your despair.

STELLA: It's a really awful feeling.

ME: How long has this been pulling at you?

STELLA: It comes and goes…

ME: What's the main thought that keeps circling around your head that sponsors your awful feeling?

STELLA: I can't see how I can ever have love in my life again…

ME: Well, just because you can't see **how** doesn't mean it can't happen…

STELLA: But, I can't even imagine it!

ME: Ah! Let's work on loosening up your imagination. You know that if you can

	imagine it, see it, dream it, believe it — it is possible to manifest it?
STELLA:	Help me see it. I know if I can bring myself to believe it, I will be able to see it.

Stella is you…Stella is me. Stella was feeling the clock ticking. *When will I have to vacate my apartment?* She felt stuck about everything. She couldn't get herself to begin the purging process. She had stopped going out on dates. She began to worry about the plan to rent a house with her friend. *What if it doesn't work? Then what?* She was afraid to move forward with anything. She stopped writing chapters for her next book. She stopped working on her life-education program. Her longings began to feel like hopeless fantasies. Her faith about the possibilities for finding love again was teetering on shaky ground. She began to seriously doubt that there were any men out there in the world who would remotely interest her. She began to sink into feelings of despair and hopelessness.

One night, Stella had a dream. She heard a familiar voice calling her name. *"Stella…Stella!"* She awakened with a quickening of her heartbeat. The voice calling her name was very familiar. Very.

It was 3:00am and she didn't want to alarm her neighbors, so she muffled her squeal of surprise. *Paul…! It's Paul's voice!* What was Paul doing showing up in her dreams?! She hadn't thought about him for over 40 years. Paul had been her boyfriend before she met Adam. It had been 50 years since she had heard his voice call her name.

Stella had learned to take dreams seriously. She wondered, *What do I do about Paul appearing in my dreams?* Was it a fluke? A portend? A message? A sign? Her dream haunted her; Paul's voice awakened her heart. She couldn't return to sleep.

Stella got out of bed, made herself a cup of tea and googled Paul's name. He showed up everywhere online. He had done some impressive work for the government. After his retirement from government work, in his 50's, he had established his own business in the music industry.

Stella was fascinated. *He's living his dream!* she observed. She found his website and wrote down his various phone numbers. It was 4:00am — too early to call him. She returned to bed and began to recall her time with Paul when they were in their 20s. Young. Passionate. She remembered him with great fondness. As she was drifting back to sleep, her body began to vibrate, similar to her physical responses whenever she would just think about Adam and Matt. It was a delicious confirmation of her vitality.

Stella awakened after getting a few more hours of sleep. At 9:00am, she was up and dressed, sipping her breakfast coffee. She decided to call Paul. After she entered the numbers and the phone began to ring, she felt her pulse quicken.

"MSL Studios...this is tech support...." It was Paul's voice! The same voice she had heard calling her name in the middle of the night.

"Paul...this is Stella...."

A long pause: "Stella...Stella? — Is that really you? — Are you still singing?"

Stella explained that she stumbled across his website, and because she had family near him, she thought it might be interesting to meet in person, after being apart for 50 years.

He was enthusiastic about the idea of meeting. "I'd love that!"

They agreed to find a date that would work for them both. Stella was feeling 25 again.

29

What You Seek...

Be realistic: plan for a miracle

— OSHO

STELLA:	I know that he is seeking me…
ME:	Yes…as Rumi says, "What you seek is seeking you."
STELLA:	I had a dream that he appeared magically out of nowhere.
ME:	Why do I have a strange feeling that he's actually nearby?
STELLA:	I've got this clear memory of him, as if I've known him before.

Stella is you…Stella is me. Stella was on fire about Paul. She believed that the dream she had was some kind of sign. The sound of his voice awakened her energy. After she called him, and they had their brief conversation, Stella continued to think about Paul, feeling an eerie incredulity at having actually reconnected with him and heard him say that he would "love to see" her.

She was replaying how he spoke her name. What she heard was a sweet tenderness in his voice…much like it had been 50 years earlier. His voice: the vibration of his voice was traveling throughout her body, streaming memories of their three years together in her youth. His voice — the memory of his words that ended their relationship so long ago — "I can't trust you..." She had been foolish, and Paul was unforgiving. His resolve to end it was unshakable, despite his parents intervening to attempt a reconciliation.

Stella had never forgotten him. Now, 50 years later, they were anticipating meeting in person once again.

In all her recent recitations of qualities she was seeking in a partner, she realized after that brief conversation, and her research about him online, that it was a man like Paul she was seeking: a partner who is passionate about his work and loves his life. A man who is healthy and vigorous, stable yet wild. A partner who is his own man, open-minded and a lifelong learner. Yes. Stella was clear about what she was seeking.

30

Frustration

*When you love, you are open and in an energy of
allowing the loving energy to flow freely. When you
fear losing love – or not getting it – you are closed
and constricted. Tight. Love cannot flow freely in an
energy of fear. Love requires you to be vulnerable.
Being vulnerable is being courageous. What can come
from being vulnerable and courageous? Everything.*

— Sheila Pearl

STELLA:	I'm so frustrated! Why doesn't he call me?!?!
ME:	What's your frustration about?
STELLA:	I'm afraid he doesn't want what I want…
ME:	And his not calling you, yet, leads you to think what?
STELLA:	He isn't as interested in getting together with me as I am…
ME:	Perhaps he's still catching up with the shock of hearing your voice…

Stella is you…Stella is me. Stella was intent on meeting Paul in person, following her phone call to him. He seemed interested in seeing her. She offered to meet him in person, explaining that she had family near him and could combine a family visit with one to him.

"I'd love to see you!" he declared. "When are you coming down?" The first date she offered, corresponding with the weekend her granddaughter was graduating from college, he had plans to be away.

The second date she offered, which was the weekend of a family wedding, Paul moaned "Oh…! I have plans to visit family upstate; let me see if I can change the date. Give me your phone number…I'll call you when I know if that date in June will work…"

The time was approaching. No call from Paul. Stella called him a few days before her planned visit. "I'm working on it…I should know by tomorrow. I'll call you."

Two days passed. Each day Stella was tempted to call him while holding back. She reminded herself, "I told him I didn't need to know until Thursday…"

It was still early Thursday. She was feeling the frustration. She was feeling the fear. She wanted to know. Yet she wanted him to be the one to call her, to say, "I've worked it out…come on down…I'm looking forward to seeing you again!"

Stella watched herself battle her two voices: *If it's meant to be it will be…* and *I can't stand the frustration of not knowing!* Stella wrestled with her fear, looking at her phone every ten minutes. *Do I call now…or do I wait for him to call?*

Stella waited…

31

Risking

The baby birds gripping the branch of the tree, the mother bird urging them to jump off, cry to their mother: "What if I fall?" and their mother replies: "Oh, my darling, what if you fly?"

— Erin Hanson

STELLA:	I'm scared! What if I get hurt?
ME:	And what if you don't?
STELLA:	I'm afraid to take that chance.
ME:	You fascinate me…
STELLA:	What's so fascinating?
ME:	You're looking for a guarantee.
STELLA:	What's wrong with that?
ME:	Nothing — if you're buying a car.

Stella is you…Stella is me. Stella was afraid of moving forward in meeting Paul until she had some reassurance that she wouldn't get hurt. Stella's challenge was to step into the unknown, to get comfortable with uncertainty. She reminded herself of her teacher's words: "If you want guarantees, you don't want life." If she was looking for a guarantee — she wasn't really looking for real life.

Stella had been spoiled by Adam, who saw her from across a crowded room and decided he was instantly in love with her. It felt like a fantasy. It doesn't usually work that way. She was fantasizing that Paul would call back and invite her visit. She was facing the ultimate uncertainty. Her clients would once again provide the mirror she needed to face herself, as she helped them see one another.

Stella's client couple, Joan and Evan, had gone through significant conflicts in their past love lives. Now in their mid-50s, both divorced, with grown children, they brought a bushel of past hurts and disappointments to their new connection. Both were afraid of being hurt again. Both were being cautious and brought guarded willingness to be totally open and vulnerable.

Stella was reflecting on how to support their growth. She remembered her own leap of faith with Adam as they were forging their young love:

> *"How do I know I can trust you? I know you've been unfaithful to others...." Stella challenged Adam.*
>
> *He looked at her and remained silent for a few seconds. "You don't. It's a matter of faith. It's not me you need to trust; it's yourself."*

Stella heard Adam's voice echo in her mind, *"It's not me you need to trust; it's yourself,"* and she savored it.

Stella realized that the magic ingredient for any couple learning to love one another was the capacity to trust in self first. She knew that self-love was essential for *Big Love* — the *Big Love* that embraced vulnerability fostered courage and compassion. Everything else would flow from that. It would be like a bird sitting on a branch being afraid the branch would break…forgetting that it had wings to fly. It doesn't matter if the branch broke; it matters more that the bird can fly.

When Joan and Evan walked in for their session, Stella sensed a tension. Her chest began to tighten up; she was tuning into their energy and felt the tension between them. She asked her higher self for the right question to begin their conversation.

"Which one of you wants to tell me about the role fear has been playing in your latest conflict?" They both started to laugh.

"I'm afraid he's going to dump me because I'm so difficult" Joan blurted out as she was laughing at herself.

Evan took her hand and moved closer to her on the sofa. "I'm afraid I don't satisfy her enough and she'll find someone else."

Because this was an ongoing theme, the three of them had learned to have a sense of humor about their conflicts and challenges.

"So…imagine how liberating it would be for each of you if you could believe that you are each delicious, sexy, and perfectly imperfect just the way you are?" Stella explored with Joan and Evan the role their fears were playing in creating obstacles to trusting and relaxing into their connection. Stella reminded them: "If each of you trusted in your wings, and stopped worrying about the branch breaking, you could actually enjoy being with each other."

Stella listened to her own guidance for her clients. It had been three months since she had been in contact with Paul. She was feeling her fear of rejection. Perhaps it would be easier if she just left it alone, if she took her cue from his silence, if she assumed that Paul just wasn't interested in meeting her. She could understand that from his perspective, he could be thinking, *What do I need from her after all these years?*

Nonetheless, Stella consulted her higher self, and decided to seriously consider going out on that limb.

32

Giving Up

Being in love is being present — if you want to be in love, stay in the moment. Let it flow naturally. The problems begin when we try to force something, hold onto something, grip and grab as if gripping would assure a loving relationship. Ha! The moment we get sucked in by fear, love can't flow or grow.

— Sheila Pearl

STELLA:	What's the use of my trying anymore?
ME:	What's the use of giving up?
STELLA:	It's so hard…so much work!
ME:	What's the point in having time, talent, and passion if you don't use it?
STELLA:	How can I be sure it will be worth my efforts?
ME:	Life isn't about the destination…it's about the journey.

Stella is you…Stella is me. Her reconnection with Paul ignited Stella's energy. She began to write again. She opened her heart to possibilities. She was excited about her big move and was taking baby steps going through her belongings and making lists of things to let go of and things to take.

Just when she had re-established momentum and re-engaged with her passionate energy, her voices of fear began to shout at her, "Don't get too excited…you could get disappointed. Slow down."

But the energy would not listen. It brought up relentless creativity. Stella was creating like she had never done before; she was designing a new life-education program for her coaching clients. She was writing her second book for her *Ageless & Sexy* series. She was envisioning having a loving relationship with a partner who matched her energy. She was filled with excitement.

She was also being distracted by the voices of fear: her fearful voice urged her to stop before she began. Her passionate voice of excitement urged her to take daily steps in the direction of her dream. She continued to shout back at fear: "Thanks for sharing!" as she was more consistently working on her projects and gathering the courage to contact Paul once again. As she took action, she noticed that she was feeling different inside: she was finding courage and imagination she didn't know was there.

Each day, Stella set aside time to write. Every two or three weeks, she met with members of her team to talk about ideas and plan her next steps. The key for her was action: to take action daily. Something, no matter how small: every step opened the pathway to the next idea, the next opportunity, the next possibility. Every word she wrote would lead her to the next. The tyranny of the empty page became her daily exercise in excitement about possibilities. "I have a new idea!" became her new diet, her response to feeling like giving up.

Being in love with her life was her choice; whether or not she would be in love again with that special person was not entirely up to her, although she was willing to take the first step.

Just as Nachshon discovered when he was the first to put his foot into the waters of the Sea of Reeds leading the way for the

Children of Israel to begin their journey to freedom, the path opens to you when you take the first step.

33

Your Mess Is Your Message

The obstacle is the path.

— Zen Proverb

STELLA:	I can't believe I've been so short-sighted and irresponsible!
ME:	What can you do about it?
STELLA:	I can't turn back the clock, can't undo the damage…
ME:	What can you learn from what you now see as mistakes or wrong turns?
STELLA:	I feel like giving up!
ME:	That sounds like a knee-jerk reaction to beating up on yourself?
STELLA:	Why does life have to be so hard?

Stella is you…Stella is me. Stella was brought face-to-face with the painful consequences of choices she made and didn't make earlier in her life. She was often so blinded by self-flagellation, she was having difficulty seeing anything but gloom and doom ahead of her.

Her client Wanda became Stella's mirror; as she was coaching Wanda, Stella awakened herself.

"What are you feeling right now?" Stella asked Wanda, who was staring off into space.

"Like I want to push everyone away from me…like I just want to climb into a hole and disappear."

Stella understood what Wanda was talking about, since she had walked down the same path many times and was walking that path currently as well. "Let yourself stay there as long as you need to be there. It's part of your journey to feel the emptiness, the despair and the guilt for all the ways you've judged yourself as 'messing up.'"

Stella and Wanda had a conversation about the mess: all the ways each of them had messed things up. They shared stories back and forth about the magnitude of misfires, false starts, screw-ups, and self-defeating patterns of behavior which had brought them both to moments of wanting to give up and back up. Their deep conversation included laughter and tears. Silence and shouting.

Wanda discovered, as they were connecting the dots together: "Is it possible that I could never have become who I am today without all the ways I messed up my life?"

Stella nodded as she hugged Wanda. "How do you think you could have developed your inner strength and resilience without all the turmoil you've lived through, my dearest?"

Stella looked in the mirror after Wanda left her office. She smiled at herself as she whispered at her reflection: "How else could you know your own depth unless you had fallen into that deep pit so many times…?"

34

Imposter

*When you love yourself with all your imperfections
and quirks, you are positioned to also really love
others who are as perfectly imperfect as you are.*

— Sheila Pearl

STELLA: I'm terrified they will find out I'm an
            imposter!

ME: I'm wondering what you mean by
            imposter?

STELLA: I'm a fake. A phony. I'm not really what
            people think I am.

ME: I'm wondering how you know what other
            people think of you.

STELLA: I want people to see me as perfect... Perfect
            in what I do. That I'm the consummate
            professional. That I'm competent and on
            top of things.

ME: Wow! That's a tall order to fill...

STELLA: And a heavy weight to carry...

ME: What do you think will happen when
            people see the truth?

STELLA: I could lose my job, my friends won't love
            me, people will look at me with disgust.

ME: Those are interesting thoughts. What if they
                       are not remotely true? What if people will
                       actually be relieved to learn that you're
                       human, just like them?

Stella is you...Stella is me. Stella had lived decades of her life believing she had to be a high achiever and perfect to get the job, to get the guy, to get respect from others.

Then she learned about the Big Lie. She learned that she had been believing the Big Lie since she was a child. She had been believing that she wasn't enough, that she had to pretend to be perfect. She had lived in perpetual fear that other people would discover she was an imposter. Then she hit the wall. She collapsed under the pressure.

She began to confess to others closest to her that she was not perfect, that she didn't have all the answers, and that she lived with fear she didn't want to admit, lest she be seen as weak.

One by one, her friends thanked her for opening up, for being vulnerable and transparent with them. They each shared with her that they felt closer to her, because she was being real. Stella began to teach others how to open up and be real with their loved ones and friends.

When Joan had hit her own wall and was hospitalized for depression, she called Stella when she was being discharged, saying, "I'm ready for you to help me fall in love with myself..."

Stella was humbled by Joan's trust in her. "I'm sending you a quote to think about. See you Monday at noon."

Joan found this quote in her emails:

> *"I have to be vulnerable by letting people know that I fall all the time. But for me going through depression was one of those places that as soon as I say that to a group of people, the entire conversation changes. They open up in a completely different way. And they realize that I'm being real, I'm not just talking about science, I'm not just talking about something that's 'Be happy all the time and everything will work out great.' We're talking about 'How do you construct happiness when it's not easy' and I've been in that place."* — Shawn Achor

"What's the most joyful experience you've had today?"

Joan sipped her tea, thinking about the question. "Hmm…my son called this morning to check in on me, saying that he wanted to have dinner with me tomorrow night. That made my heart Dance!"

Stella and Joan began their journey of discovery and affirmation of the truth and the lies of life. "I'm not enough" is the Big Lie. "I am *Big Love*" is the truth.

35

What Is Real Love?

My heart is open. I allow my love to flow freely. I
love myself. I love others and others love me.

— Louise Hay

STELLA:	I had this strong unwavering feeling that we reconnected for a reason!
ME:	And what did you think that reason was?
STELLA:	Why would we magically reconnect after decades if not for love?
ME:	And what was the message love had for you?
STELLA:	I had this overwhelming feeling that the love we had long ago would bring us together again in a very significant way.
ME:	Define "significant..."

Stella is you...Stella is me. Stella believed that hearing Paul's voice calling her name in a dream was an invitation. When she found Paul after Googling his name, then magically reconnected with him, she had the strong feeling and belief that they were "destined" to get together again after decades of being apart.

Paul had sounded enthusiastic about meeting her when he responded "Of course! I'd love to see you again!" Yet when they attempted to find a time that worked for them to meet, Paul had conflicts. He had asked for her phone number, saying he'd get back to her about a specific weekend they discussed. He didn't call her back. She wondered. She waited. Was she totally off base? Was she imagining the whole thing? Was her dream about Paul just a fluke, leading to her discovery of him, for no particular reason at all?

Stella noticed her own thoughts and feelings ebb and flow, rise and fall during the weeks between her initial dream about him and their phone conversations. Thoughts like:

I have this feeling of deep soul connection with him; I'm convinced he came to me in my dream for a reason!

After all these years, I can imagine picking up where we left off 50 years ago...I have a feeling of deep love for him, as if no time ever passed.

Perhaps I heard his voice calling my name in my dream because he's looking for me...

Maybe he's not calling me back because there's a part of him that doesn't want to see me again.
Maybe he's hesitating on getting together with me because he's afraid to open that door...

I'm afraid I'm just making this whole thing up...and his silence is telling me what I don't want to hear; he's not interested in reconnecting.

Stella sat observing her collection of thoughts and emotions swirling around her body and mind. She chose to wonder instead:

I wonder what the gifts are and could be that Paul came to me in my dream.

I wonder how I can apply my feelings of deep love for Paul at this moment.

Stella reminded herself of the power of surrender…the power of letting go of things she could not control. She began to *kythe* with Paul. She sent him pure love. She sent him her intention of loving him regardless of the outcome she wanted. Yes, she wanted to see him. However, if he didn't want to see her, she realized she only wanted to be with people who couldn't wait to be with her. She didn't want to be in a situation in which she was either trying to convince or persuade someone to meet with her.

Stella wanted Paul to be happy and healthy in his life. She had thought there was a possibility that in reconnecting, they would bring joy and love to one another. If not, she wished him joy and love in the remainder of his life without her.

She continued her *kythe*: *"I wish for you joy and love all the days of your life."*

Stella's heart remained open. She stopped looking at her phone, checking to see if Paul had called her. She surrendered to what was so at that moment in time. She smiled at her open heart, feeling at ease as she sent Paul love without an agenda.

36

Risking Vulnerability

Hold still. Stay there. Tease back the layers. You are in the space between your comfort zone and infinity. You want to hide. Not be seen. Not be open. Not be vulnerable. But you have to. There are two ways to do this — soft and gentle or fast and hard. Both will get you to the other side, if you let them.

— Jeanette LeBlanc

STELLA: I'm afraid of taking another chance.
ME: What's at stake?
STELLA: I might make a mistake.
ME: What else?
STELLA: I might get hurt.
ME: What else?
STELLA: I might be disappointed.
ME: If you want guarantees, you don't want life…
STELLA: I just don't want pain.
ME: No pain, no gain. Yes, you might fall down and make mistakes. And you might learn something. Yes, you might get hurt, and you might experience triumph. Yes, you might be disappointed, and you might also be surprised.

Stella is you…Stella is me. Stella was feeling her own fragility, not sure if she wanted to venture outside her comfort zone and risk rejection, or hurt, or disappointment. That was her conundrum. She wanted that beautiful relationship without risking the pain of failure or disappointment. Her challenge was to risk, to choose to be vulnerable.

Stella reminded Wanda, "When we love someone, it's a gift. The other may or may not accept our gift. The gift to ourselves is that we opened our hearts to love."

Wanda listened, as tears welled up. "It's true…there are times I want to hide and not be seen. Maybe he feels the same way. It's not easy to be vulnerable. It's not easy for me to keep my heart open, when I'm feeling frightened. Maybe I'll choose the soft and gentle way…"

Stella was inspired by Wanda's courage and vulnerability.

It had been three months of silence from Paul, which she was hearing as his rejection of her. She decided to step aside from making assumptions and being stopped by her fear of his rejecting her, and she called him.

He answered, "Hi, I'm so glad you're calling! I lost your number. When are you coming down again?"

37

Magical Reunion

*I choose each day to be the conscious director of my
own movie. I always retain my inner power and
vision for the outcome I choose to experience.*

— Debra Oakland

STELLA:	I'm floating on the wings of our magical reunion, and I'm feeling the emptiness of uncertainty about what's next…
ME:	How about treating "what's next" as an exciting adventure?
STELLA:	I would feel better if we had a specific plan.
ME:	You already have a specific plan…
STELLA:	I wouldn't exactly call it a plan. Certainly not a specific plan.
ME:	Sounds like you want the whole script written out, now.

Stella is you…Stella is me. Stella risked: After nearly three months of silence from Paul, she decided to take a leap, to risk vulnerability, and to call him. He was cheerful and asked how she was doing.

She answered with calm, "I'm fine and enjoying life. I was wondering…when you didn't call me back to arrange a visit, I wasn't sure if you were interested in reconnecting."

Paul laughed and quickly reassured her: "I lost your phone number! I'm so glad you called…"

Stella giggled to herself as she reminded him that she knew him well. "I see you're still the absent-minded professor and mad-scientist."

He laughed. "You've got me right…so when are you coming down again?"

She explained that she could come when she wanted to visit and could plan a trip that would accommodate his schedule. "Would you prefer to meet during the week?"

Paul paused for a moment then agreed: "It would actually be easier that way…sometimes my weekends get jammed up."

So they made a plan. He insisted on coming to pick her up at her family's home. The day finally arrived when she would meet Paul for lunch.

After not seeing one another for 50 years, Stella was wondering how best to greet him: should she hug him? Wait and take his lead? She was feeling like a nervous school girl.

Paul finally arrived at her family's home. Her son-in-law answered the door, they shook hands as Paul fixed his eyes on Stella standing nearby and walked over to her, kissing her on the cheek. Paul also met Stella's two grandchildren who were there. Paul was relaxed and engaging with her family; Stella felt a warmth for him as they all had a brief conversation.

As Paul was helping Stella into his car, he looked at her hair and said, "I think I had better close the sunroof to protect your hairdo…"

She was touched by his thoughtfulness. "Yes…my hairdo is a bit more fragile than it was 50 years ago." They laughed as he closed the door.

Once he got into the driver's seat, he announced, "I want to introduce you to my new love: Thibaudet. A brilliant French pianist. I've been listening to him play Ravel as I drove down here."

Stella was already in heaven: Paul loved the music she loved, and he was sharing his "new love." How perfect! He had chosen a little Middle-Eastern cafe for lunch and conversation. It was magical for her. Their conversation was animated as each shared what they had been doing with their lives. Stella was feeling a reminiscent twinge of sweetness rush through her heart.

Paul had been Stella's chief cheerleader when she was an aspiring opera singer. "Would you be interested in hearing my operatic demo recording?" she offered.

"Of course!" he replied. "Do you have a CD with you?"

When they got into the car after lunch, Stella reached into her purse and pulled out the CD, handing it to him.

"I'm very excited…" he said as he placed it into his CD player. The first aria began. After the first few notes, Paul exclaimed, "Whoa…! That's not the voice I remember! You really worked hard! I'm impressed!"

Stella was thrilled.

Paul insisted on listening to a few tracks, before walking Stella to her door.

"You don't have to listen to the whole thing now…it's yours."

As they were saying goodbye, Paul said, "This was a great idea. Let's meet again soon." Then they kissed. For her, the kiss was reminiscent of a sweetness they had once shared. It was tender.

An hour later, Paul called, "I listened to the remainder of your CD as I was driving back home; I'm inspired. Just wanted you to know. Thank you!"

For Stella, the aftermath of that reunion was a mixture of exhilaration and pain. She wanted more. She wanted it immediately. It wasn't happening the way she wanted. She wanted specific follow-up plans, like the following weekend or month. He was vague: "We will arrange to meet again soon...either down here again, or up in your area. We'll make it happen."

Stella felt the challenge of uncertainty. She felt the pain of impatience. She was being intentional about her self-talk, *I trust all will unfold in the perfect way for us both...*

She recoiled from the thought that she was being invited by this situation to trust. To trust the process. To trust the Universe. To trust him. To trust herself.

Her little voice reassured her, "It was no coincidence that you reconnected...trust that this is all happening in the perfect time and place for you."

Stella made an entry in her journal after she returned from their reunion lunch:

> *It's not easy to be patient and trust the Universe when love has filled my heart and I want to share, to hug and kiss, to connect and to expand the magic of one moment into the next.*

Stella's invitation was to trust...to lean into the process...and to remind herself how she accomplished the first miracle.

38

The Lock Box

Every bee that brings the honey
Needs a sting to be complete
And we all must learn to taste the bitter with the
sweet.

— Naomi Shemer

STELLA:	Imagine my surprise to see a lock box on my door!
ME:	What?!
STELLA:	A lock box…the bank locked me out of my apartment.
ME:	Can they do that?
STELLA:	Yes…they can…and they did.

Stella is you…Stella is me. Stella could no longer avoid the reality of her financial difficulties. The terms of her reverse mortgage were that if she was in default by failure to pay her real estate taxes or maintenance she would be given the opportunity to buy back the property or vacate the property. Once the bank secured the property by changing the locks and putting a lock box on her front door, it was the bank's procedure to give her 30 days to vacate her apartment.

When Stella arrived at her apartment at 11:00pm at night, locked out and facing the lock box on her door, she began to laugh.

She surprised herself by breaking into laughter at her situation. She went to her office to sleep and called her attorney in the morning. Her attorney contacted the bank and arranged for Stella to receive the combination to the lock box, so she could gain entrance to her apartment. The bank confirmed that Stella would be given 30 days to vacate.

Until that day, Stella was convinced and firmly believed that she needed a minimum of 90 days in order to purge and pack her accumulation of belongings. 90 days was not an option any longer. Her plan had been to rent a house with a friend; her challenge was to find a house to rent and do what was necessary to move within a month.

She was facing the impossible. She had been saying to herself, *It's impossible to do this!* She changed her self-talk: *How can I get this done?* Within two days, her friend found a house to rent and they paid their deposit for the rental. They were in high gear, excited and overwhelmed.

Stella posted on Facebook that she was in the midst of purging and packing for her move. Within two days, she had over a dozen people who had volunteered to help her. She created a schedule for her helpers to come over to her apartment to help her purge her belongings between clients. They would help throw out the items she couldn't give away and didn't want to keep and begin to distribute donations and pack the items she decided to keep.

While she maintained her coaching practice, she was organizing her team who helped her by throwing out hundreds of bags of trash, donating dozens of boxes of books to churches, the book exchange, and synagogues, and bringing dozens of bags of clothing and household items to the Goodwill and Habitat for Humanity's ReStore.

Stella was going through emotional turbulence as she excavated 45 years of memorabilia, choosing which of her 100 framed art pieces to keep and which to give away or sell; deciding which of her hundreds of ceramic and crystal treasures to keep or give away; deciding which of her furniture to keep or give away. With each item she considered giving away, she was feeling a pain in her heart. Piece by piece, she practiced "letting go" as if a spiritual exercise. She had close friends by her side as she said goodbye to her various treasures, often holding her as she cried in the midst of her releasing process.

Each day of her purging and packing became an emotional, physical, and spiritual practice of release.

39

Sweet Dreams

Where is the perfect place to start?
You'll never know until you get to the end.

— Crissism

STELLA:	I listened to my little voice and it was magic!
ME:	What was magic?
STELLA:	He called me, and we talked for nearly an hour!
ME:	Anything else magical?
STELLA:	Yes. We are meeting again next month.

Stella is you...Stella is me. Stella was in the midst of a great uncertainty in her life. Her first meeting with Paul was magical. Sweet. Connecting. Affectionate. Yet she heard nothing from him in three weeks. She was apprehensive about seeming pushy.

Stella had established a practice of *kything* and writing love letters to him on her notepad, which she never sent; they were all purely intuitive. They were her way of connecting with him heart-to-heart both intuitively and spiritually, while remaining "quiet" and not pushing him.

Three weeks after their reunion meeting, Stella was in the middle of *kything* with him and writing her love letter on her notepad, when she heard her little voice whisper, "Call him." Really? Call him? So, she did.

It was 1:00pm and although Stella thought it was risky to call him in the middle of the day, she followed her intuitive message. She called.

He answered the phone and with a hurried voice said, "I'll call you back!"

Stella understood that he was in the middle of something he couldn't interrupt, yet had answered the phone, knowing it was her. She waited. At first, she thought he might return her call in a few minutes, and even kept her phone with her when she went to the bathroom. After a couple of hours, she let go.

As Stella was sipping her evening tea at 9:40pm, Paul called her back. "Sorry about earlier today...I was in the middle of a sound experiment."

Stella understood. He was busy with his work. Stella laughed to herself: "He's the mad scientist and absent-minded professor. Get used to it!"

In their 90-minute conversation, their banter was substantive. He talked about his mother and added, "When we get together next time, remind me to tell you stories about my mother in my recording studio!"

Stella was thrilled. He was already thinking about what he wanted to share when they got together again.

They made plans for their next meeting. Stella asked, "Is it ok with you that I remind you about our plans and even be a gentle nudge?"

He laughed and agreed that he needed to be reminded. "Please do...you've got me right!"

*When we get together next time…*was a song that kept playing over and over again. She loved the melody! Stella had very sweet dreams that night.

40

Mahler

No reason is needed for loving.

— Paulo Coelho

STELLA:	Any man who appreciates Mahler is my kind of guy!
ME:	Do you know anyone like that?
STELLA:	Only one…

Stella is you…Stella is me. Stella was discovering how much she and Paul had in common: even more than had been the case 50 years before. What they had in common was their mutual love of music…many kinds of music.

It was very early in their relationship-building journey and Stella wasn't sure how their connection would evolve. She had decided to listen to her little intuitive voice of wisdom as she stepped into their process of discovery.

She and Paul had agreed to a second lunch visit. In the meantime, he was busy with work and Stella was busy both with work and preparing to move out of her apartment into a house. The task was daunting for her, so she turned to music as her companion and support. She had a special passion for all things Mahler. It was something she had shared with her husband for 32 years. She missed sharing her passion.

As she was purging her belongings, throwing out and giving away clothing, books and CDs, she found some of her Mahler CDs and began to play them. She felt the impulse to share with Paul, so texted him a YouTube link to one of her favorites.

A day later, she received a text from Paul: "I find Bernstein's rendition of this Mahler too schmaltzy for my taste...try this one." He included the link to another recording conducted by Sir Adrian Boult. Paul also included a link to some vocal music by Mahler which he thought Stella would enjoy. "Here's a beautiful vocal and symphonic rendition of his songs..."

How could Paul have known that those were among Stella's favorite songs, which she had sung herself many times?

Stella was literally tingling with joy. Her heart was dancing. No other man in her life than her husband had ever appreciated Mahler. She was thrilled that Paul not only appreciated Mahler but had a keenly discerning ear for the differences in conductors of Mahler's music.

Stella felt a certainty that their connection was on its way to growing into some form of sweet substance and she was relishing the taste.

41

Thanksgiving

*Open your mind. Allow your feelings to be expressed,
to be pushed out, and your heart will neither break
nor burst, but be a free-flowing channel of the life
energy in your soul.*

— Neale Donald Walsch

STELLA: My heart is so full, I can't stand it!
ME: Tell me more...
STELLA: Our second visit was even more magical
            than the first!
ME: Tell me more...
STELLA: He shared stories about his mother whom I
            loved...
ME: And...?
STELLA: We fed one another at the table...
ME: And...?
STELLA: And...he put his arm around me as he
            walked me to the door, and then kissed me
            like he didn't want to let me go.

Stella is you...Stella is me. Stella was following her intuition, opening her heart, and feeling the exhilaration and the fear mixed and churning in the big bowl of uncertainty which was ahead of her. After 50 years apart, Paul had re-entered her life and her heart.

She wanted to spend more time with him, while he seemed content to spend two hours sharing lunch and conversation. She wanted him to make plans for getting together again, while he seemed relieved leaving it to her to arrange.

A few days before her second visit with Paul, Stella had completed the big move out of her apartment into a house she was renting with a friend. The six weeks between her first and second visits with Paul had been a challenging and busy; she was feeling proud of herself for purging 45 years of accumulated belongings and reducing her possessions to a fraction of what she had accumulated. She was also deeply grateful for all the friends who had helped her pack up her belongings and move. Stella was feeling excited about her new adventure in living with a friend and creating a home together. Stella's heart was filled with gratitude for all her blessings.

"I'm running late; see you at about 1:30," was Paul's message. Stella was amused as she observed that Paul was still the same "absent-minded professor" he was when she was dating him 50 years earlier.

Paul arrived to pick her up at her family's home at 2:15. He had decided on taking Stella to one of his favorite restaurants nearby, where they enjoyed sharing a big bowl of mussels and a shrimp salad. Paul fed Stella the best mussels, scooping up the delicious soup as he reached across the table with each succulent bite. She took sweet delight in watching how much he was enjoying his lunch.

As they were enjoying their culinary pleasures, Paul shared funny stories of how his mother would give her candid feedback to the musicians during recording sessions.

"I loved your mother...she was such a zesty lady!" Stella reminisced.

Then they began talking about Israeli politics, and Stella could feel a deep tension begin to simmer. Paul suggested she read a book he recommended, before they went any deeper into that arena. Stella was willing; she felt challenged. Paul was inspiring her to stretch. It had been what she loved about him in her youth, and 50 years later, it remained an endearing quality for her.

After lunch, Paul ushered Stella out of the restaurant, took her hand, then put his arm around her as they walked toward the car. Back at her family's home, Paul escorted her to the door, walking slowly with his arm around her, holding her close to him as she put her head on his shoulder — like two old friends cuddling. Standing at the door, Stella felt a kiss coming toward her. Paul pulled her close to him and kissed her ardently.

"I so enjoy being with you!" Stella whispered.

He kissed her again. "Yes. We do have fun, don't we?" he smiled.

Stella was floating in the divine flow as she entered the house.

42

After Shock

Get comfortable with uncertainty. Possibility resides here.

— Sue Urda

STELLA: I was standing at the front door in shock with my hand still holding the knob, dripping with blood!

ME: What happened?

STELLA: The dog bit my hand…

ME: My goodness! Then what?

STELLA: My friend rushed me to the emergency room.

ME: And…?

STELLA: And I had over 20 stitches in my hand and fingers. It was deep.

ME: And…?

STELLA: That was the beginning of the end…and a new beginning.

Stella is you…Stella is me. Something shocking happened. After the shock, Stella asked the most important question: "What's next?"

Stella suddenly found herself facing her worst nightmare: she had only been living in her new household for a few days; she was neither feeling "at home" nor was she feeling safe. She had not yet been introduced to her friend's dog — her only contact with the dog had been the night he bit her hand as she was entering the house. As the days passed, Stella was feeling both puzzled by not meeting the dog, and consequently feeling increasingly unsafe. The new living arrangement didn't feel like home.

During the holidays, while Stella was away with her family, she texted her friend that she needed to feel safe in the house — and until she could feel safe with the dog, she was not willing to stay at the house.

Her friend responded, "This isn't working…it's best you seek alternative living arrangements."

Stella was in shock: they had barely moved into the house together, she had not yet met the dog, and her friend was telling her "This isn't working…" Was this a dream? A nightmare? Was it real? Was she kidding? Where would she go? What were her options?

Stella's good friend Orah immediately offered Stella a place to stay while she figured out her next steps. Because everything was in a state of uncertainty, Stella had no idea what furniture she would be able to use as she moved forward. It was clear to her that she could not afford to move her piano and dining room set into storage: she would need to sell or give away these treasures. Habitat for Humanity doesn't take beds or sofa beds, so she would have to give away or throw away these items. Her bedroom furniture was 45 years old and had decades of wear and tear; she decided to give away or throw away her bedroom set. A few smaller items including her wingback chair and bookcase she decided to keep and put into storage.

Friends went with Stella to the house to help her pack up and remove her personal belongings, clothing, dishes, crystal, books and kitchen supplies. All of these items she put into storage.

Stella needed to find a home for her most precious treasures: her baby-grand piano, her dining room table and chairs, and her china closets. She wanted to know her treasures would be in a good home. She placed ads online and made calls to people who bought and sold used furniture. It was a frustrating process; Stella had a feeling of great urgency because she wanted all of her belongings out of the house as soon as possible.

As Stella was letting go of her personal belongings, she felt lighter — even liberated — from releasing the heavy weight of her big furniture. She realized that this expanded the options for her next step because she wouldn't have to accommodate so much big furniture. Sixteen years earlier, Stella needed to shop for the right space to accommodate her furniture and chose her condominium apartment for its expansive wall space and a place for her piano. With fewer belongings, she would have more choices of spaces: smaller, simpler, and more affordable at this stage of her life.

Despite the shocking unexpected outcome of her move into the house, Stella felt excited about her future, despite uncertainty…or perhaps because of uncertainty. She said to herself with a smile, *I'm traveling light!*

43

Birthday Present

If you live the questions, life will move you into the
answers.

— Deepak Chopra

STELLA:	My little voice whispered, "He needs you to call him."
ME:	And…?
STELLA:	The first two times I heard that message, I held off on calling him.
ME:	Then…?
STELLA:	In the middle of my birthday celebration, I heard the message whisper again. So…I called him.
ME:	And…???
STELLA:	He answered, "It looks good."

Stella is you…Stella is me. Stella was floating in a sea of uncertainty. After two magical lunch visits with Paul, she risked inviting a third meeting. She had suffered the silence. He hadn't yet responded to her invite for her third visit.

A day passed…then the second day whizzed by.

Three days after her call, she was in the midst of her birthday celebration. Her good friend Carole asked what she wanted for her birthday. "I want to hear Paul's voice."

As soon as Stella stated her birthday wish, her little voice whispered: "Call him now."

Stella called him; he answered. As soon as he heard her voice, he asked, "Could I call you back? ...I got your message, and it looks like I can work it out."

Stella got her wish. She could hear in his voice that he wanted to work it out. It sounded like he wanted to see her again soon. His voice reflected the sweet gentle connection they were creating.

Stella's birthday was special for her; Carole had prepared her favorite meal — rack of lamb, medium rare. She had wrapped up a few birthday trinkets, all thoughtful and loving examples of Carole's quality of friendship. "I love it when you're here, Stella! You are such a gift to me!" was Carole's affirmation of her appreciation for Stella.

It was easy for Stella to return the accolades. "You know, Carole...you are a perfect example of *Big Love*: you are open, generous, and loving without an agenda. I love you dearly! I'm deeply grateful for our friendship."

Stella and Carole enjoyed the delicious meal which Carole prepared. They laughed together as they shared stories of their lives, their adventures, and escapades. Carole wasn't as much of a night owl as Stella, so she retired for the night early leaving Stella to enjoy her own company.

Stella's practice on each of her birthdays was to acknowledge her many blessings in her journal. She entered the following list of her many birthday presents:

> *I'm deeply grateful for my good health and good friends,*
> *for my talents and my beautiful memories,*
> *for my challenges and my bitter moments of pain and disappointment,*
> *for my losses and my gains,*

for my mistakes and my ability to be resilient,
for my triumphs and my ability to be humble,
for those who have hurt and disappointed me,
for my love of myself, and
for the many people who trust me with their souls.

44

Giving It Up

Love is the only true freedom from attachment. When
you love everything, you are attached to nothing.

— Mikhail Naimy

STELLA: I'm giving it up.
ME: What are you giving up?
STELLA: Believing that Paul is my last resort.
ME: Hmmm…where did this come from?
STELLA: Loving myself.
ME: I don't understand.
STELLA: If he doesn't see me, or appreciate me, he's
             not "The One" and I'm willing to believe
             there's someone else looking for me.

Stella is you…Stella is me. Stella thought that perhaps she had
that dream and that Paul had come back into her life as "The One"
she desired to experience. She was seeing Kismet in their
rediscovery of one another; yet Paul was not as communicative as
Stella wanted him to be. She wanted reciprocity. She wanted to
know that Paul shared her enthusiasm for exploring a relationship.
    She talked to herself, saying, *I know I'm a special woman. I've got*
so much to share and give. I want to be with a man who sees me and
acknowledges my value to him. Anything less is a waste of my time!

Although the first two meetings with Paul were enjoyable and the goodbye hugs and kisses were exceedingly sweet, Paul was silent for weeks in between their visits, without connecting. Stella struggled with the silence, telling herself not to take Paul's silence personally.

It had been nearly two weeks since their brief conversation on her birthday, in which he asked, "Can I call you back?" She didn't understand his silence.

Her little voice whispered, "Use the silence for your own growth...listen into the silence."

She kept listening.

"I can't control what he feels or wants with me...I need to give up insisting on anything at all."

Stella observed herself feeling a sadness as she repeated the mantra, "I'm giving up my attachment to him..." Her tears were listening to his silence.

45

Look What Happened

Waiting for someone else to change is the long road to happiness.

— Byron Katie

STELLA: Look what happened after I gave it up!
ME: Tell me...
STELLA: Paul called me the next day!
ME: And...?
STELLA: We DID meet for lunch again... after all.
ME: And...?
STELLA: I think I'm learning more about both of us.

Stella is you...Stella is me. Stella had wrestled with her demons of attachment, struggling mightily to overcome the pain of being attached to the outcome of anything at all. Her challenge was to accept her reconnection with Paul for exactly what it was naturally designed to be; to allow the process of discovery to take its divine place in her life rather than push or insist on anything at all.

Easier said than done. Stella was feeling the clock tick. *Life is short!* she kept saying to herself, feeling the inner tug of impatience and the discomfort of uncertainty. For Stella, she would feel ever-so-much more at ease if Paul moved toward her more quickly, if he gave her the experience that he was as eager to see her again as she was to see him.

Just as she gave up the belief that Paul was the last resort, letting go of her insistence that he be a certain way at a certain time, he surprised her and called back: "Hi...this is Paul...I'll be home all evening...call me back." He was calling to let her know that he could see her for a third visit.

"Yes, either Wednesday or Thursday will work for me."

They agreed on 2:00 since Stella was driving down that morning.

As Stella was sitting with Paul during their lunch visit, she began to feel a familiar loneliness: she had been there before with other men she had dated since Adam passed. She recognized that empty feeling of irrelevance, wondering if for Paul, she was simply another of his enthusiastic audience, listening to his interesting stories. It occurred to Stella that Paul was very content with his life just the way it was; content to meet with her occasionally for lunch; content to keep their connection simple and sweet.

Paul alluded to returning to one of the restaurants they had visited previously when she made her next visit, and she observed herself jumping to conclusions like a giddy school girl — *Yes! He wants to see me again!* — making it mean something more than it likely meant for him.

As Stella was driving back home from her visit with Paul, she reflected on the benefits of "giving it up" — she was feeling at ease with whatever developed. She was able to be more present to Paul and herself, in the exchange, since she wasn't preoccupied with *What does this mean?* or *Where is this going?* She understood that it was going exactly where it was designed to go. She was grateful for having reconnected with Paul, keeping her heart open for the divine flow of energy to take them where they decided together to go.

46

This Isn't Working

Whenever a relationship or situation isn't working
for one person — it isn't working for either one.

— Sheila Pearl

STELLA: Those words pierced my heart and I felt broken.

ME: What words pierced your heart?

STELLA: "This isn't working…"

ME: If something isn't working for one person in a relationship or situation, it isn't working for either one. It seems to me that these words are simply feedback…

STELLA: They don't land as feedback…they land as a knife in my heart.

ME: Hmm…give yourself some space to reflect and lean into what you're feeling…

STELLA: You're telling me to smile and breathe deeply aren't you?

ME: Yes…

Stella is you…Stella is me. Stella was in the middle of a difficult situation which resembled others in her life: she was feeling dismissed and disregarded in ways that were familiar, only the packaging of the situation was different.

She remembered the night her temple board voted not to renew her contract, when she thought the board would be voting on her salary increase.

When the president called to inform her of the vote, Stella was incredulous and hurt: "What happened?"

"This isn't working."

The president's cryptic remark hit her in the heart. She couldn't believe her ears. It didn't make any sense.

It took Stella several months to get to the heart of the matter — which had less to do with her than with finances — and to heal from the assault to her heart.

Stella's head also spun after seeing her housemate's text, "This isn't working…"

Stella received a call from a client who said he was in crisis. Stella heard the tears in Jason's voice: "She said it's over; it isn't working. I'm heartbroken!"

Stella listened as Jason told his story.

"I'm feeling your heartbreak along with you," Stella said as she leaned into Jason's sadness, breathing deeply as her way of energetically opening her heart to Jason in his time of grieving. "Give yourself some time to feel everything you're feeling right now. Don't judge it. Lean into the pain. Smile. Breathe deeply. Smile again and continue to breathe deeply. "

Stella knew that Jason had been having his own misgivings about his relationship with Amy. "When something isn't working for one — it isn't working for either one," she would remind Jason.

Jason had been stubbornly determined to make things work with Amy, pushing aside his own misgivings.

When Amy announced that "this isn't working," Jason could only hear the message that he was being dismissed and thrown away. He couldn't see that he also felt some relief as well; relief from having to continue to pretend he had no misgivings. Amy had taken him off the hook.

Stella recognized her own painful and disappointing situation in Jason's heartbreak. "This isn't working" is feedback more than judgment, although it usually feels like rejection and a knife in the heart.

Stella told Jason her story with the Temple Board:

> *Although I had been unhappy at the Temple for many reasons and had been planning to leave and begin my own coaching practice, it hurt my feelings that they dismissed me so easily. It was from that situation that I learned when something isn't working for one side, it isn't working for either side.*

As Stella looked back on her aborted living situation, she realized that she felt a strange tension and coldness from the moment she had moved into the house — never feeling that she was "home."

After the dog bite, tensions escalated, and Stella could see that there was a no-win dynamic festering. As she reflected on her brief stay in that house, Stella felt a relief that she was on the other side of that arrangement, as painful and expensive as that experience was for her.

47

Twilight Zone

Embrace uncertainty. Some of the most beautiful
chapters in our lives won't have a title until much
later.

— Bob Goff

STELLA:	I feel like I'm in the Twilight Zone…
ME:	Hmm — sounds mysterious.
STELLA:	Yes. Life is mysterious, and my head is spinning…
ME:	What's your story?
STELLA:	I'm interested in getting to the other side of the story.
ME:	How do you do that?
STELLA:	You've taught me well: I ask my higher self the right question; "How can I make this mess a blessing?"
ME:	Yes, you define the quality of your life by asking the right questions.

Stella is you…Stella is me. Stella's new living situation didn't work out. Her challenge was to explore alternative living arrangements.

The situation forced Stella to look at herself in ways she had previously avoided. She was asking, "Who am I now…? What do I want now…? What does *home* look like to me now?"

Then, as she was feeling the surges of anxiety rushing through her body, she asked the most important question: "How can I make this mess a blessing?" It felt like a big mess, a big conundrum, a big puzzle piece that life was inviting her to put together.

Stella was in uncharted territory. She was swimming in the sea of uncertainty, reminding herself that *this is where possibilities reside.* She laughed at herself as she observed her own calm in the midst of the storm.

She could see more clearly than ever that her mess was her message.

48

Safe Haven

You are breathtakingly beautiful. Exquisite. Extraordinary. There is no one like you. And you are here at this time for a specific purpose and as part of a divine plan. Now, love yourself for who you are, in your flawlessly perfect state of imperfection. Because when you love yourself, you set yourself free to receive love and to give love away to others.

— Daniel Nielsen

STELLA: I'm surrounded by love!

ME: You sound surprised.

STELLA: Not surprised; deeply grateful.

ME: Well, in the midst of your mess, you have blessings?

STELLA: Many. I have the blessings of a safe haven.

Stella is you...Stella is me. Stella needed a safe haven while she regained her balance, removed her belongings from the house, and saved money for yet another move.

Good friends immediately offered her a room in their home where she could stay while she decided what to do next. "You will have to treat your room like a hotel, since we don't have a closet and there's no storage space," her good friend Orah explained. "We love you and you are a part of our family. We want you to feel totally at home."

When Stella arrived with her bag packed with a few essentials, she saw that Orah and her husband had gone shopping for a 5-drawer dresser that fit nicely into Orah's office/guest room. Orah had also purchased a coat tree and put out some hangers so Stella could hang a few articles of clothing. There was a bathroom next to the guest room which was virtually Stella's own private bathroom with a large shower. Orah gave her one of the extra garage-door openers; Stella had easy access to the house through the garage which allowed her into the finished downstairs where she slept.

For everyone in Orah's family, and for Stella, it was an easy transition. Stella would enter and leave the house from downstairs, without disturbing anyone else in the family. The family dog, Sophie, often greeted Stella when she came home and sometimes slept in her room. Her safe haven felt cozy, welcoming, and comfortable.

During the following few weeks, Stella and her friends made regular trips to retrieve her belongings from the other house while Stella decided what to do with her furniture and secured a storage unit. She found the contrast of living in a house for over a month which never felt like home versus the secure comfort of staying with Orah and her family informative.

Stella began to recognize the many ways she was experiencing a "safe haven": her office where she spent the majority of her time was her home base; her good friends, her spiritual community, and various tribes were connective tissue; and her team of coaches and mentors provided additional emotional and spiritual sustenance. The living situation that didn't work became less and less a story that commanded center stage for Stella. Instead she focused mostly on the many ways she was surrounded by love, by support, and by possibilities.

Stella understood that she was experiencing a big shock, a big disappointment, and a big impact on her financially and emotionally since packing up to leave her apartment, then moving into the rental house, and finally removing her belongings from the house again. She had learned the power of surrender.

She asked for support and help from her friends and communities. She allowed herself to cry and laugh, as she sang songs of joy to the Universe for all the love that surrounded her. *I love you Stella...* she would say to herself in the mirror every morning, reminding herself that she was a work in progress.

49

I'm Bleeding

How people treat you is their karma; how you react is yours.

— Wayne Dyer

STELLA: So, as I'm bleeding in the midst of this
            awful mess, tell me what I'm supposed to
            see in this "mirror"!

ME: Reflect on other times in your life you felt a
            similar emotion...

STELLA: You mean like "irrelevant" or "invisible"
            like when my father abandoned me? Or
            when my stepchildren acted as if I was
            dead?!?!

ME: Yes. That's what I mean.

STELLA: What's the "mirror" about here?

ME: What did you learn from the mirror your
            father and stepchildren provided to you?

STELLA: It took a while for me to see it...and
            eventually I learned that the mirror they
            provided showed me the illusion and not
            the truth of who I was.

ME: Yes. And what else?

STELLA: I learned how to NOT take their behavior
            towards me personally.

ME: Bingo.

Stella is you...Stella is me. Stella was in shock as she was recovering from her tumultuous series of moves, the unexpected dismissal, and the feelings of hurt and disappointment. She felt a deep disappointment in someone she had believed was her friend.

She asked herself, *How can I move forward out of this shocking situation?*

It was Stella's practice to own her circumstances and to seek understanding where there was conflict. She found herself in a no-win situation (something difficult for Stella to accept) in which simply walking away appeared to be the only healthy option for her.

Stella's coach asked, "When else did you feel this way?"

Stella recognized those feelings of being disposable, invisible, irrelevant and alone.

"What do you know is real about who you are?"

Stella had learned that she was a valuable human being — anything but irrelevant. Stella had learned to recognize the difference between the truth and the illusion of who she was. Throughout her life, she had been in relationships that challenged her to ask *Who am I?* and *What is true about me and what is false?* or *What is illusion and what is truth?*

When her father had abandoned her, she spent decades of her life taking his behavior personally, believing that something must have been wrong with her to explain her father's abandonment of her. It took decades of self-exploration for Stella to understand that her father's lack of capacity to love her was not about her at all.

Likewise, when Adam's teenagers came to live with Stella and Adam as they began their marriage, Stella was once again challenged not to take her stepchildren's behavior personally. They didn't want Stella in their lives, so they treated her as if she wasn't

184

there. She had a choice: to allow herself to feel irrelevant and invisible, or to understand that she was relevant and a loving human being regardless of how others treated her.

When her congregation dismissed her, didn't renew her contract, and told her "it wasn't working" she took it very personally. Until she realized that the Temple Board's action that affected her life was more about finances than about her. She understood that she was anything but irrelevant and being dismissed opened the doors for her to begin her coaching practice.

Stella looked in the mirror and repeated her daily mantra: *I love you Stella. You are here to be a source of love to yourself first and to others. Remember what mama taught you: those who are most unlovable need the most love; just love them!*

Stella got dressed and mapped out her strategy for reconstructing the big mess in her life. She was proceeding one smile and deep breath at a time.

50

No Address

Behind all seen things lies something vaster;
everything is but a path, a portal or a window
opening on something other than itself.

— Antoine de Saint-Exupéry

STELLA:	I've never been homeless before…
ME:	How are you feeling about it?
STELLA:	Strange — liberated — like I can fly in many different directions…
ME:	What do you make "homeless" mean to you?
STELLA:	I'm learning to redefine "home" as people rather than a place.

Stella is you…Stella is me. Stella never expected to be homeless. She had walked away from her condo which was in foreclosure. She had moved into a house with a friend, looking forward to creating a home. It didn't work. She found a safe haven with good friends who offered her a room in their house while she decided what to do next.

It was the middle of the night and Stella felt the room whirling around as she started to get up to go to the bathroom. She practically fell off the toilet, as her dizziness persisted. She recognized anxiety in her body and began to breathe slowly and deeply. She carefully walked back to her bed from the bathroom, as the room continued to whirl around her.

What was her body telling her? Stella asked herself, *Who am I now that I have no home? What do I do with all my stuff that has no place to go?*

Her head was spinning, and it felt like the room was spinning. She continued to breathe deeply and notice her thoughts. She reminded herself to smile. Although it seemed totally counter intuitive to smile, she knew that smiling was her way of telling her brain that she was in charge.

A few seconds after she began to smile in the midst of her deep breathing, Stella noticed her heart beat slowed down, and the room stood still.

How do I feel being here with my friends?

She felt at home. Her friends were loving and protective. She realized that for her, "home" was the quality of friendships she had created. Having some safe haven was reassuring and grounding; even more important for Stella was being at home with a few of her best friends.

While sorting out her various choices for a more long-term living arrangement, Stella was enjoying the adventure of exploring herself as well as enjoying her friends. Now that she no longer owned her apartment, she was like a free bird, flying high above the trees.

51

Catharsis

Grief is something we integrate. We don't get over it.

— Sheila Pearl

STELLA:	It was a strange catharsis, watching two men reduce my furniture to rubble...
ME:	Tell me more about the catharsis.
STELLA:	I'm not sure how to describe it; I'm witnessing two guys destroy my bedroom furniture and throw my old bed on the trash heap, and I felt lighter...
ME:	It sounds like a burial...from dust to dust...
STELLA:	Maybe that's it. Letting go of all attachment is liberating.

Stella is you...Stella is me. Stella was letting go of many of her belongings: furniture and other items which had been a part of her environment for decades. She was choosing to return many of her material possessions to dust. "From dust to dust" was her way of putting her experience of letting go in perspective.

She reminded herself, *Everything has a beginning and an end. Each of us comes from dust and each of us returns to dust.*

In Stella's career as a spiritual leader, she had officiated at countless funeral services, supporting her congregants as they lovingly laid to rest their loved ones. Stella had buried her own children, her parents, her grandparents, her friends, and her husband. She was an experienced warrior in accepting the fact of death and appreciating the ritual of burial, in which the physical reality of "dust to dust" becomes visceral and embedded in one's emotional DNA.

The "GOT JUNK" truck arrived. It cost Stella $700 a truck-load to have her furniture taken away. The only way they could fit everything into one truck load was to break down all the furniture, literally demolishing each piece. She decided to stand in the driveway to witness the destruction, much as she would stand at the edge of the grave as the dirt is shoveled in to fill it up.

As her bedroom furniture was being demolished in front of her, Stella chose to make this a sacred "passing" for her: she reviewed her life history with her bedroom furniture she and Adam had purchased 45 years before its destruction.

She remembered purchasing the large ivory lacquered shelving unit which had held her books and objects d'arte in Adam's and her her large Townhouse.

Three tall bookcases and the cherry entertainment unit also had to go. The coffee table, sewing-machine desk and large ottoman had to go.

Then she took a deep breath as she let go of the bed she purchased after Adam passed. It had been 13 years and she needed a new bed. It was time to let this bed go... It was time to let almost everything go.

As the workers filled the truck to the top, closing it up before driving to the dump, Stella silently said a blessing for all of her furniture which had served her and her family for decades.

This was a time of profound transition for her, as she blessed the energy of her belongings being returned to the earth.

190

52

Getting Better

As we walk through our journey, we break. Our
hearts break, our bodies break, our spirit breaks.
That's what happens. How we put ourselves together
with our broken pieces is our genius and our art of
living.
It's a beautiful thing to behold!

— Sheila Pearl

STELLA:	It doesn't get any better…
ME:	It sounds like deep satisfaction.
STELLA:	I thought I needed little intimate nibble kisses…
ME:	And…?
STELLA:	I discovered that those nibble kisses are more about a sweet energetic heart-connection than the physical intimacy.
ME:	And…?
STELLA:	Being together with loving friends for an evening of connection and celebration of life is **so** sweet!
ME:	And…?
STELLA:	And deeply satisfying!
ME:	Like nibble kisses…?
STELLA:	Maybe even more…

Stella is you…Stella is me. Stella was longing for an experience of intimacy akin to what she had enjoyed with Adam and Matt. She often felt a despair of never having that sweet connection again. In between visits with Paul, not knowing where they were going, she was riding the wave of uncertainty.

As Stella was reeling from the changes taking place in her life, her good friends in Florida invited her for a visit. "Come and enjoy some warm weather. Get away and clear your head!" She agreed.

During planning and packing for her trip to Florida, the realities of her temporary living situation became humorously apparent; she needed to visit her storage unit, take out her travel bag, and find summer clothing and sandals. Temperatures in the 20's in New York, she was packing for sunny Florida with temperatures in the 70's.

Stella was looking forward to her visit to Florida as she packed her suitcase. Her friends Cat and Donna were among her closest friends and she missed them deeply.

The flights to Tampa from New York turned out to be frustrating: the outgoing flight was delayed due to icy conditions. Consequently, she missed her connecting flight in Philadelphia. She called Cat to let her know she would be on the next flight, two hours later.

Cat met Stella at the airport in Tampa. It was a welcome sight to see her dear friend! When she entered Cat's home, she saw a bouquet of her favorite white roses on the table.

"Are these for me?" Stella asked.

"Of course they are! And I also have your favorite rack of lamb ready for our dinner tonight."

Wow! Stella felt surrounded by love and thoughtfulness. It was just the beginning of her visit with her friends. When Donna joined them later for dinner, she was carrying her famous stuffed mushrooms. It was a feast of friendship and yummy food.

Donna took Stella home with her, where she would be staying during her visit. Both Donna and Cat had planned some special events for Stella. Two nights after Stella arrived, Donna had organized a dinner party, inviting some of her close friends to join Cat and Stella. The table was artfully set as if for royalty. Donna prepared her specialty "Captain's Chicken" recipe, which she knew was one of Stella's favorites.

As the six friends were enjoying their feast in Donna's home, Stella looked around and felt the close circle of loving connection. She thought to herself, *It doesn't get any better than this!* What a sweet evening of satisfying engagement. She was sated.

The last night of Stella's visit, Cat and Donna surprised Stella with tickets to the Sarasota Symphony performing a concert of her favorite composers: Ravel, Chopin and Debussy.

As Stella sat in the concert hall feeling the music wash over her like a warm shower of love, she smiled and felt the tears fall down her cheeks: *This is what sweet love feels like....* Her heart was overflowing. *This is oneness. This is* Big Love.

Once Stella returned to New York from her Florida visit with Cat and Donna, she was feeling the truth of *Big Love* in her life more than ever before. She understood on a visceral level the truth of her soul movement in her life: her friends were mirrors for Stella reflecting back to her that she was loving and loved. She was feeling the energy of love surrounding her, as she returned to her arena of uncertainty.

She was determined to say "YES!" to all of the options available to her for affordable housing. Before her visit to Florida, she was saying "NO!" to options like relocating to Florida. During her visit, she surprised her friends when she agreed to carefully consider relocating to Florida as one of her options. Cat and Donna were hopeful that Stella might eventually live near them.

Stella had a brainstorming meeting with members of her team. "What is most important to me?" was a central question they explored together.

Stella was clear that she wanted to keep her office, maintain her coaching practice, and build her speaking career. Stella's connections with friends and communities were central to her emotional and spiritual health: she had spent decades building relationships within her various friends and groups. She understood the role that maintaining those relationships would play in her longevity and creativity. She also realized that she needed housing in a situation that was simple, safe, and affordable. Whereas she had once said "NO!" to senior housing, she made application for several of the affordable senior communities in her area. While she was on the waiting list, she continued to explore all options available to her.

It had been two months since Stella and Paul had their last visit. It had been three months since Stella had spent quality time with her granddaughter. It was time for another visit to Baltimore.

She checked with her granddaughter for her availability for a dinner visit together. They decided on a date.

One week before her trip to Baltimore, Stella called Paul to let him know when she was driving down, letting him know she would be available for lunch if he was interested.

Three days later, Paul called Stella to confirm he could meet her.

Stella was delighted, excited, heartened, and yet calm. Stella surprised herself with her "calm" during her conversation with Paul.

She smiled when he said, "I look forward to seeing you."

She thought to herself, *I love you, too…*

53

Surprises

The most valuable possession you can own is an open heart. The most powerful weapon you can be is an instrument of peace.

— Carlos Santana

STELLA: My life is just chock full of surprises!
ME: That sounds like you're excited.
STELLA: Yes. Excited...and scared.
ME: Tell me more.
STELLA: I'm excited about all the beautiful, loving,
            miraculous experiences I've been having in
            the midst of my big mess!
ME: And you're scared about...?
STELLA: I'm afraid of all the uncertainty and
            uncharted territory ahead of me.
ME: Buckle up...

Stella is you...Stella is me. Stella was between addresses. She stopped thinking of herself as "homeless" and instead acknowledged she simply had "no address" other than her Safe Haven address with friends, or her office. In fact, she knew she would not have to fear ever being homeless, because so many friends loved her.

She was at a crossroads, exploring choices about her next chapter: did she want to live with "family of choice" or would she opt to live alone? Would she stay where her office was in New York, or relocate to a warmer climate?

Looking back over an inventory of her recent life, Stella surprised herself.

During a period of 90 days, she accomplished what she had once believed was impossible. She moved out of her apartment into a house within 30 days with the help of a team of angels.

Then, after living in the house only 36 days, in a state of shock, with the help and support of her angels, she managed to move her belongings out of the house within six weeks, putting some essential belongings into storage and letting go of 90% of her furniture.

She had learned that what she believed about anything really did make a difference. In spite of the uncertainty during those 90 days, Stella managed to maintain her good health and vitality. She was thriving in the midst of the messy transitions, serving her clients, and completing the manuscript for her next book

In the midst of a turbulent 180-degree upending in her living situation, she learned that miracles and blessings often come from the ashes of destruction.

Stella made a point to keep her sense of humor. She gave a speech at her Toastmasters Club in which she began by saying: "You make plans...and God laughs!" She described herself as "traveling light" since giving away her baby grand piano and dining room set, plus destroying other large pieces of furniture.

Her options for living space or relocating anywhere she might choose were enhanced by her letting go of most of her belongings.

Among Stella's greatest pleasures in giving away her treasures was shipping her two Henredon China Closets to her grandson.

Her Henredon dining room table and chairs were with a good friend in town. Her baby-grand piano was with a friend nearby. She could visit her furniture from time to time. Stella was doing a happy dance knowing her treasures were safely with family and friends, enjoying good homes.

As she was celebrating giving away her treasures, she thought of Heidi who came to take her sofa bed, crying, "I never thought I'd be in this situation…thank you so much!"

Stella reassured Heidi, "We're all in this cosmic stew together…I never thought I'd be here either, and now I'm happy to give you my sofa!"

Once Stella had finally removed all of her belongings from the house, she looked forward to her next visit to Baltimore. She was excited to see Paul and her granddaughter again.

As she pulled into the carport at her family's home, she heard a voice message from Paul: "I was wondering if I could come earlier to pick you up for lunch."

Stella called Paul to let him know she had just arrived, and he could come any time.

"See you soon!" She could hear the smile in his voice. She had time to visit with her son-in-law and freshen up before Paul arrived.

When Paul arrived, he rang the doorbell and Stella's son-in-law answered, greeting Paul. As Stella was getting up from her chair in the family room, Paul walked toward her with a broad grin and holding out his arms as they hugged and kissed. Her heart was wide open.

There was some interesting magic in their fourth visit: it was comfortable, in the midst of the uncertainty for her. Stella was leaning into the discovery process. Paul was a fascinating man and she was enjoying the gradual pace of becoming reacquainted after so many decades apart. He was both familiar and uncharted territory. She was intrigued by him, while feeling comfortable as they shared another meal together, feeding one another and laughing together.

"We do have a good time, don't we?" Paul whispered in her ear as he kissed her goodbye. He was full of surprises.

She looked forward to the next time. Her heart remained wide open.

54

Moving Forward

It hurts to love wide open
stretching the muscles that feel
as if they are made of wet plaster,
then of blunt knives, then
of sharp knives.

— Marge Piercy

STELLA:	I'm facing the great bowl of Jell-O…
ME:	You mean the great uncertainty?
STELLA:	Yes…the great uncertainty.
ME:	What are you feeling right now as you face it?
STELLA:	Excitement…and terror.
ME:	Tell me first about the terror.
STELLA:	All those voices of doubt and limitation are shouting at me.
ME:	What do you do about those voices?
STELLA:	I turn down the volume.

Stella is you…Stella is me. Stella felt like she was swimming in a big bowl of Jell-O. It felt uncertain, unstable, unknown, like she was entering the dark and suspenseful Tunnels of Love in Coney Island.

For over 14 years, her coaching practice had been the epitome of uncertainty: she would never know where the next call would come from, what her monthly income would be, how long a client would opt to stay with her, who would show up or cancel an appointment on any given day. She had learned to ride the wave of uncertainty, almost like an exciting ride at the amusement park.

That was all important information for Stella. Her coach would reassure her, "Look at how you have thrived in your practice throughout the roller-coaster ride of uncertainty..."

At her monthly Grace spiritual study day, her friends were helping her clarify alternatives for her next living situation. They read a portion of Rumi's poem:

> *The breezes at dawn have secrets to tell you*
> *Don't go back to sleep!*
> *You must ask for what you really want,*
> *Don't go back to sleep!*
> *People are going back and forth*
> *across the door sill where the two worlds touch,*
> *The door is round and open*
> *Don't go back to sleep!*

Stella's community supported her in looking at her options, including the ones to which Stella had originally said "*NO! NO! NO!*"

What was she resisting? What was she insisting on? Stella understood that "what you resist persists," so agreed to go through the process.

Stella had been resisting living alone. She wanted to live with family or "family of choice." She had been insisting on living with others, while also insisting that living alone was dangerous — not safe for her.

In the process of digging deeper beneath her insistence and resistance, Stella excavated her deep sadness in losing family and her home no longer being what it once was. She had sunk into the pit of resignation and hopelessness, rather than remaining open to the possibilities of living alone which could be liberating rather than frightening.

When Stella began to explore her options, living alone in affordable housing available to people over 55 became more attractive to her. Having a one-bedroom apartment which was in a secure building with easy and safe access became more appealing to her.

She visited the various sites and completed her application; she was officially on the waiting list. It could be two months or longer. She didn't know. It was all uncertain.

In the meantime, Stella clarified for herself what was most important for her: she wanted to keep her office, maintain her coaching practice, and continue to pursue her speaking career.

She also wanted to continue to pursue the possibilities of having a significant love relationship. How would that look? She was revising her vision. It was uncertain. Was Paul a possibility? It was uncertain.

Stella, who had lived alone many years, had learned that living with other people gets complicated. She wanted simple. Stella needed her solitude and privacy. Living with other people could create more static for her than ease. She had learned that she could have sleepovers with friends and community, to satisfy her need for connection and intimacy.

It could be both/and rather than either/or: she could enjoy the togetherness with friends on an occasional basis, while affording herself the solitude and privacy she craved on an ongoing basis. The idea of living alone was no longer on the "*NO! NO! NO!*" list. It became an idea that commanded a resounding "*YES! YES! YES!*" It was a simple shift in perspective.

Stella's most recent lunch visit with Paul was a revelation: it became clear to her that he enjoyed her company and was simply very content with his life and willing to let things flow.

Was that a mirror for her? Wasn't she also very content with her own life, alongside enjoying his company? Was it possible that she could get comfortable with the uncertainty of their future together, allowing things to flow?

YES! YES! YES! she answered herself.

Epilogue

Attention is love, what we must give
children, mothers, fathers, pets,
our friends, the news, the woes of others.
What we want to change, we curse and then
pick up a tool. Bless whatever you can
with eyes and hands and tongue. If you
can't bless it, get ready to make it new.

— Marge Piercy

Over 50 years ago, while I was completing my bachelor's degrees at UC Berkeley, I attended a lecture in my Religion class which I have not forgotten; a guest lecturer, talking about belief in God.

The Rabbi asked us, "Who here believes in God?" Most of the hands in the auditorium of 500 students went up. Then he asked, "How do I know you believe in God?"

Hands went up, volunteering a variety of answers including "I'm a good person" or "I attend church" or "I study the Bible."

He looked around the theater. "No! You're not even close!" You could hear a pin drop. His pause was especially pregnant as he looked into our eyes. "When you pay attention to your friend, to your parent, to your pet, to your plants." *Paying attention* was his point.

The Rabbi's point was profound: he was instructing us in the fundamental law of the Universe. *Where you put your attention will expand.*

205

His message was that we were each co-creators with God; that how we pay attention to ourselves, our friends, our loved ones, our pets, our communities, our environment would be proof of our belief in Life itself. He was equating God with Life; God with Love.

When Stephen Levine writes "Hell is wishing that life be anything other than what it is," he is reminding each of us that Life Is — it isn't fair or unfair. It just is. It's not easy to remember that, I know. However, when I *do* remember the truth of that, and stop resisting what is, and remember to lean into the inevitable uncertainties that are inherent in life itself, I can begin to breathe more easily and lighten up. When I can lighten up, I can open myself up to the next moment of possibilities that are right in front of my face, if I would just pay attention!

I can't tell you how many people I talk with daily who will say things like "it isn't easy being me!" When my friends or clients will laugh at themselves — much like I can laugh at myself — life just gets easier.

Step by step, as I walk this path of my beautiful messy life, I'm finding that I'm getting increasingly *more* comfortable with uncertainty. I didn't say I'm comfortable with uncertainty: I said increasingly *more* comfortable. And...I didn't say it stays that way; it's a dance of leaning in and pushing back, resisting and resting...until...

Until...I resist less, rest into enthusiasm; resist less, rest into fun; resist less, rest into more creativity and vitality. This can be so for you, as well. I know for me, as I get more comfortable with the uncertainties of my life — the financial, the personal, the physical — I open the channels for my own energy to flow more easily, for my vision to be clearer, for my mind to be free to imagine possibilities instead of conjuring reasons to be afraid.

In a novel by Tayari Jones, *An American Marriage,* the essence of what I see as *Big Love* is expressed in this letter from a husband to his wife:

> *"At night, if I concentrate, I can touch your body with my mind. I wonder if you can feel it in your sleep. It is a shame that it took me being locked up, stripped of everything that I ever cared about, for me to realize that it is possible to touch someone without touching them. I can make myself feel closer to you than I felt when we were actually lying in bed next to each other. I wake up in the morning exhausted because it takes a lot out of me to leave my body like that. I know it sounds crazy, but I'm asking you to try it. Please try to touch me with your mind. Let me see how it feels."*

When I read this segment, I couldn't imagine a more perfect expression of *oneness* and the phenomena of transcending the physical to the spiritual.

I know that I'm not alone in my longings; it is our human nature that longs to experience something of ourselves that is bigger than the physical, bigger than the mental, bigger than the often-limited confines of what romantic love has become for many. What most of us long for is to experience the expanse of being human, to be *in love* with ourselves and others, without it being about possession or attachment.

I know that I am no different from you: I long for a bliss that occurs when I allow myself to push through my fears, when I can say to fear with a sense of humor, "Thanks for sharing!" as I step into one risky moment after another, feeling my power as I summon forth my courage, as I choose to replace my judgment of myself and others with ultimate compassion and empathy.

Magic is what happens when I allow my imagination to fly and my heart to remain open to possibilities; it is my open heart that opens a pathway to my creativity.

Brene Brown's now-famous quote, "Vulnerability is the birthplace of belonging, community, and creativity," rings true throughout the messages in my story here and is a central theme in the work I do daily with clients.

As I keep my heart open to possibilities and lean into uncertainty, I continue to understand a deeper longing that I have — the longing of our human condition to experience our own authenticity, our own magnificence, our own sexiness. We can experience that connection with our own essence in our most intimate relationships; we can also experience that bliss as we acknowledge our own essential selves in our creativity.

Big Love is what I experience when I risk singing the high note, knowing that to do so I could crack or squeak, or my voice could ring out with luster and brilliance.

Big Love is what I experience when I risk getting a rejection as I invite a former boyfriend for a lunch visit and he answers me with "I'd love to see you!"

Big Love is what I experience when I write another manuscript, send it to my editor, and am willing to hear "this isn't hitting the mark yet" and willingly, enthusiastically revise and revise again until I do hit the mark.

The Magic of Big Love is about allowing the uncertainties of life to open you up to a new awareness of your big dreams, your big heart and your big possibilities.

— *Sheila Pearl*

About the Author

Sheila Pearl - a seasoned clinical social worker, life coach, bereavement counselor and family therapist - was married for 32 years before becoming widowed. It was then she began her unexpected sexual, spiritual, sensual and magical renaissance. She is actively dating, seeking her next life partner, while also passionately engaged in her career as a relationship coach and an international speaker. Sheila is dedicated to coaching men and women around the globe who are motivated to develop and expand loving relationships with themselves and others.

Former opera singer and teacher, Sheila is a lifelong learner and gatherer of wisdom. She has earned seven bachelor's degrees from the University of California at Berkeley: in English Literature, Music Performance, Speech & Drama, Religion, Philosophy, Sociology and Psychology. She completed the Certification Program with the Hebrew Union College for Cantorial Studies, having served two congregations in New Jersey and New York for over 20 years as cantor and educator. She is an ordained non-denominational minister and wedding officiant. She earned her master's degree in clinical social work from Yeshiva University's Wurzweiler School of Social Work and was certified as a life coach by the Empowerment Training Institute, founded by David Gershon and Gail Straub, co-authors of *The Art of Empowerment*. As a family therapist, she trained with Virginia Satir in family systems theory and practice. She studied with Neale Donald Walsch, serving as staff coach for the Life Skills Program as part of the Conversations with God Foundation for five years. Since retiring as cantor and educator in 2004, she has had a busy private practice in relationship and life transitions coaching.

Sheila is the author of *Still Life: A Spiritual Guidebook for Family Caregivers;* and co-author in the bestselling book "Pearls of Wisdom: 30 inspirational ideas for your best life now" with Jack Canfield and Marci Shimoff, in *Living Passionately: 21 People Who Found their Purpose and How You Can Too,* and in *Wake Up Women! Be Happy Healthy & Wealthy* with Arielle Ford and 50 other coaches. Sheila's first book in the *Ageless & Sexy* series, *The Magic of Sensuality – A Love Story,* became an Amazon bestseller in October 2015.

Find *Ageless & Sexy* books at AgelessAndSexyBooks.com; visit Sheila at www.sheilapearl.com; follow Sheila on Facebook at www.Facebook.com/SheilaPearl; email Sheila anytime at info@SheilaPearl.com; or call her at 845-542-6057 and leave a message if needed.